Current Practice in Health Sciences Librarianship

Alison Bunting

Editor-in-Chief

Volume 2
Educational Services in Health Sciences Libraries

Edited by
Francesca Allegri

Medical Library Association
and
The Scarecrow Press, Inc.
Metuchen, N.J. & London
1995

British Library Cataloguing-in-Publication data available

Library of Congress Cataloging-in-Publication Data

Educational services in health sciences libraries / edited by
Francesca Allegri.
p. cm. — (Current practice in health sciences librarianship ; v. 2)
Includes bibliographical references (p.) and index.
ISBN 0-8108-3004-3 (acid-free paper)
1. Medical libraries—United States. 2. Library orientation—United States.
I. Allegri, F. (Francesca) II. Series.
Z675.M4E35 1995
026.61'0973—dc20 95-11863

Manufactured in the United States of America

Printed on acid-free paper

Educational Services in Health Sciences Libraries

Contents

Preface

Current Practice in Health Sciences Librarianship (CPHSL) continues the publication principles established by its predecessor, the *Handbook of Medical Library Practice,* to serve as: a general introduction to the field of health sciences librarianship for graduate students; a source of basic information and references to the literature for the Medical Library Association's (MLA) professional development and recognition program; a reference work for health sciences librarians and other information specialists, providing basic information in areas peripheral to their own expertise; and a means of documenting the state of practice of health sciences librarianship at a praticular point in time.

The decision to change the title of this venerable MLA publication is best explained by a review of the *Handbook*'s publication history. The appearance in 1942 óf the first edition of the *Handbook,* published by the American Library Association, fulfilled a long-standing goal of the MLA. As editor Janet Doe noted,

> The demand [for a Handbook] has grown keener with the passage of time, undoubtedly because of the recent rapid increase in the number of medical libraries, for half of the 315 now existing in this country have originated since 1910. To staff these libraries, workers have been enticed or commandeered from general and special libraries, from library schools, from the clerical staff of hospitals or medical schools, and from doctors' offices [1].

The second edition of the *Handbook* (1956), edited by Janet Doe and Mary Louise Marshall [2], updated the one-volume first edition, retaining, whenever possible, the original chapter authors. The preface to this volume included an apology for publication delays and noted that some of the information in the volume was written three or more years prior to publication.

Fourteen years elapsed before the third edition, the first one published by MLA, appeared in 1970. Editors Gertrude L. Annan and Jacqueline W. Felter took an entirely different approach: "The chapters are written by a new cadre of authors and differ from those of the earlier edition in substance and emphasis" [3]. Despite the expansion of the scope and coverage, the one-volume format was retained. Four consultants from different types of health sciences libraries ensured that the content took into account library practice in these settings. Publication delays continued to be a problem and were

> ...of grave concern to the editors who regret that some chapters were written several years before the volume went to press. With so many involved in the preparation of the work, unforeseen emergencies arose which prevented its production in the period scheduled [4].

Louise Darling, David Bishop, and Lois Ann Colaianni edited the fourth edition, published between 1982 and 1988. This edition included a "...shift in terminology from medical to health science libraries...in itself...indicative of the new complexity, the highly interdisciplinary nature of the fields served by these libraries" [5]. However, the title of the *Handbook* was not changed "...because of the risk of obscuring the continuity of editions" [6]. A three-volume format was chosen to: "...accommodate material on new developments, lessen the delays inherent in a mutiple-author work, and facilitate later revision..." [7]. This new approach did not, however, prevent publication delays

> ...even with a smaller number of authors per volume, the considerable time difference in submission of chapters has meant that the problem of keeping material within the volume on the same level of currancy, though reduced, has not been solved [8].

And, "...the sequential publication has resulted in problems of uneven currency in the completed work..." [9]. "A more satisfactory method for revising the Handbook in the future is now under study, as the rapid pace of change in the information field obviously requires a new approach" [10].

In 1989, the MLA Books Panel recommended that the *Handbook* be continued with the same general scope and content as the fourth edition, but that the three volumes be further divided into a series of smaller monographs, each dealing with a single subject and each with its own volume editor. An editor-in-chief, assisted by an Advisory Committee, was appointed to coordinate the publication.

The Advisory Committee determined that health sciences librarianship is changing so rapidly that the profession will be better served by publication of a series, and that the series required a new title. In this way, individual volumes can be updated as needed, without having to wait for the completion of all volumes in an edition, and the individual volumes will have a greater identity as independent books.

CPHSL will appear in eight volumes. The editors are noted below:

Volume 1: Reference and Information Services in Health Sciences Libraries, *M. Sandra Wood, editor*

Volume 2: Educational Services in Health Sciences Libraries, *Francesca Allegri, editor*

Volume 3: Information Access and Delivery in Health Sciences Libraries, *Carolyn Lipscomb, editor*

Volume 4: Collection Development and Assessment in Health Sciences Libraries, *Dottie Eakin and Daniel T. Richards*

Volume 5: Acquisitions in Health Sciences Libraries, *David Morse, editor*

Volume 6: Bibliographic Management of Information Resources in Health Sciences Libraries, *Laurie L. Thompson, editor*

Volume 7: Health Sciences Environment and Librarianship in Health Sciences Libaries, *Lucretia W. McClure, editor*

Volume 8: Administration and Management in Health Sciences Libraries, *Rick B. Forsman, editor*

The editor-in-chief is extremely fortunate in being able to tap the expertise of a group of very talented and dedicated MLA members as advisors, editors, and chapter authors. The CPHSL Advisory Committee provided valuable advice on the organization and content of CPHSL, recommended a publication plan and timetable, and assisted in the identification of editors and chapter authors.

The editors have total responsibility for the preparation for publication of their volume, including selection of authors, review of content and adherence to established style and format guidelines, and maintenance of the publication schedule. Authors were asked to include in their chapters, as applicable, the following considerations: ethics, standards, legal aspects, staffing issues and implications, differing practices as they apply to different types of libraries, research, evaluation, technology/automation, and budgeting and finance.

An extensive expert review process involved both academic and hospital librarians. Each volume includes a listing of the expert reviewers of that volume, in grateful acknowledgment of their efforts. The editor-in-chief and the editors are indebted to MLA's Managing Editor of Books, J.

Michael Homan, for selecting reviewers and coordinating their work, and for his personal suggestions on organization, content, and format.

CPHSL is co-published by the Medical Library Association and Scarecrow Press, Inc. Special thanks are due to David B. Biesel, Director of Scarecrow's Association Publishing Program, Raymond S. Naegele, MLA's Director of Financial and Administrative Services, and Kimberly S. Pierceall, MLA's Director of Communications, for their advice and assistance. The indexing expertise of Beryl Glitz provides consistent and accurate access to the content of each volume.

Alison Bunting, Editor-in-Chief
Louise M. Darling Biomedical Library
University of California, Los Angeles

References

1. Doe J, ed. Handbook of medical library practice. Chicago: American Library Association, 1942:v.

2. Doe J, Marshall, ML, eds. Handbook of medical library practice. 2nd ed. Chicago: American Library Association, 1956.

3. Annan GL, Felter JW, eds. Handbook of medical library practice. 3rd ed. Chicago: Medical Library Association, 1970:v.

4. Ibid., vii.

5. Darling L, Bishop D, Colaianni LA, eds. Handbook of medical library practice. 4th ed. vol. 1. Chicago: Medical Library Association, 1982:xi.

6. Ibid.

7. Ibid., xii.

8. Darling L, Bishop D, Colaianni LA, eds. Handbook of medical library practice. 4th ed. vol. 3. Chicago: Medical Library Association, 1988:xiv.

9. Ibid.

10. Ibid, xv.

Expert Reviewers

Holly Shipp Buchanan, Augusta, GA
Jayne C. Campbell, Baltimore, MD
Anne Fredenburg Dolan, Towson, MD
David S. Ginn, Pittsburgh, PA
Jane A. Lambremont, Asheville, NC
Nardina Nameth Mein, Detroit, MI
Rochelle L. Minchow, Irvine, CA
Beverly Renford, La Jolla, CA
Faith VanToll Ross, Chicago, IL
Phyllis Soben, Los Angeles, CA

Advisory Committee Members

Rachael K. Anderson
Director, Health Sciences Center Library
University of Arizona,
Tucson, AZ

Alison Bunting
Associate University Librarian for Sciences
Louise Darling Biomedical Library
University of California, Los Angeles
Los Angeles, CA

Dottie Eakin
Director, Medical Sciences Library
Texas A&M University
College Station, TX

Rick Forsman
Director, Denison Memorial Library
University of Colorado Health Sciences Center
Denver, CO

Ruth Holst
Director of Library Services
Medical Library
Columbia Hospital
Milwaukee, WI

J. Michael Homan
Director of Libraries
Mayo Foundation
Rochester, MN

Mary Horres
Associate University Librarian for Sciences
Biomedical Library
University of California, San Diego
La Jolla, CA

Kimberly Pierceall
Director of Communications
Medical Library Association
Chicago, IL

M. Sandra Wood
Librarian, Reference and Database Services
George T. Harrell Library
Milton S. Hershey Medical Center
Pennsylvania State University
Hershey, PA

Authors

Francesca Allegri
Training/Education Consultant
Champaign, IL

Karla Hahn
Network-based Services Manager
Welch Medical Library
Johns Hopkins University
Baltimore, MD

Abigail Hubbard
Independent Consultant
and Visiting Professor
Deparment of Management
University of Houston
Houston, TX

Nadia J. Martin
Reference/Instructional Librarian
Undergraduate Library
University of Michigan
Ann Arbor, MI

Diane G. Schwartz
Associate Director for Medical Education
Research Associate Professor of Medicine
Primary Care Resource Center
School of Medicine and Biomedical Sciences
University at Buffalo
State University of New York
Buffalo, NY

Mary Joan (M.J.) Tooey
Director, Information and Instructional Services
Health Sciences Library
University of Maryland at Baltimore
Baltimore, MD

Melanie L. Wilson
Health Sciences Librarian for Collection Management
Hardin Library for the Health Sciences
University of Iowa
Iowa City, IA

Elizabeth H. Wood
Head, Reference Section
Norris Medical Library
University of Southern California
Los Angeles, CA

Introduction

Scope

Twenty years ago, it would have been hard to imagine that educational services in health sciences libraries would grow sufficiently to deserve a volume in the Medical Library Association's handbook series. Indeed, growth has been such that it is even necessary to limit the scope of this volume. *Educational Services in Health Sciences Libraries* deals with educating library users, not library staff, with one exception: training staff who provide user education is covered in the chapter on administration. Neither does this volume deal in any depth with patient education or consumer health education. These topics are addressed in Volume 1 of this series, *Reference and Information Services in Health Sciences Libraries,* and will also be covered in *Hospital Library Management* [1].

This book follows the intent of *Current Practice in Health Sciences Librarianship* to be an introduction, an overview, and a state-of-the-art depiction of educational services in health sciences libraries. This book is not intended as a detailed, step-by-step guide to planning and implementing educational programs. Several good examples of such guides already exist [2-5].

Others have succinctly presented the highlights of the history of instructional services [6-7]. In recent years, hospital and academic librarians have continued to meet the challenges posed by key players in the arena of health care education [8]. The programs documented in the literature are numerous and innovative [9-15]. This volume summarizes what has been learned from those efforts and describes trends that will affect educational programming in the future.

Throughout this book, the term *user* designates the library user or library patron. This is consistent with prevailing usage and conforms with the other volumes in this series. The phrases *educational services* and *instructional services* denote the teaching activities of library staff. Based on the literature, the terms *information literacy, information management education,* and *bibliographic instruction* are used to label particular approaches to the health sciences librarian's teaching role [16-17]. These terms are defined in Chapters 3 and 4.

Background

Health sciences libraries have a product that is needed by all health care professionals to adequately perform their jobs: organized and accessible information. The amount of information emerging from research efforts alone makes it impractical for professionals to scan all the literature relevant to a particular interest area. Memorizing all the new facts is unrealistic. Keeping up with one's specialty by attending an annual conference and reading a few select journals is no longer possible.

Health care educators now place value on lifelong learning as an essential condition of competent professional practice. This emphasis has been paired with a need to understand how to access, organize, and manage information. In the last ten years, the librarian's role as educator has gained greater significance because of health care professionals' responses to the sheer volume of information available. Health sciences librarians have devised education programs in information management to meet health professionals' needs in this area.

In health sciences libraries, where issues of life, death, and human well-being are everyday concerns, educating users in information-seeking skills complements the provision of document delivery, reference, and other services. There is synergy among these services, which can be viewed negatively by those who become overwhelmed by diminishing resources. The mission of health sciences libraries — promoting health and improving patient care — is met when these services operate smoothly, effectively, and in cooperation. In educating users, either one-on-one or in groups, librarians not only help users find the information they need for the patient care question of the moment, but they also encourage more frequent and effective use of the library's collections, databases, and staff. Empowering users to seek information in an independent and ongoing fashion is generally recognized as the best way to prepare users for the realities of an information and computer age [18-19].

Education programs are not a substitute for the individual help that users occasionally need and receive through signs, written instructions, or regular reference services. They do, however, provide a method for users to be helped collectively, particularly when the members of the group are comfortable working together or have the same research problems, clinical questions, or class assignments. They also provide a public relations opportunity in which librarians can promote specialized products and services that may otherwise be unknown or appear so new and difficult that users avoid them. Other reasons that continue to fuel educational services are economic. Print and nonprint tools, and some group instruction, are a means to preempt routine queries. In addition, the library's image and support from users are strengthened because of the institutional contacts made in preparing and delivering educational services.

Much has been written about the information explosion, living in an information society, and the impact of technology [20-24]. The theory and methods of teaching users have evolved as librarians have grappled with the effects and implications of a changing environment. Teaching process versus tools, educating versus training, providing lifelong learning skills versus meeting an immediate need, and the librarian's role in continuing education are just a few examples of the discussions in the literature [25-29]. These debates have a rapidly changing and complex environment as their underpinning.

Since the fourth edition of the *Handbook of Medical Library Practice* [30], library educational services have been altered in response to technological advances. Card catalogs have been closed or even removed; users are doing their own searching on locally mounted systems or Compact Disk, Read-Only Memory (CD-ROM); and many libraries provide microcomputer labs with sophisticated hardware and software. Librarians are teaching users about communications software, Internet resources, electronic mail, downloading, and reprint filing.

In the process of teaching, librarians may use local area networks, CD-ROM networks, Ethernet connections, desktop publishing software, liquid crystal display (LCD) devices, or slides that are, in fact, computer graphics. Further changes that will affect educational services are increased use of optical storage, worldwide networking, electronic access to online catalogs, and electronic mail and telefacsimile (FAX) for document delivery [31-33]. As the sources of information and the ways they are accessed have become more complex and technologically sophisticated, the content and methods that librarians employ to teach users have changed accordingly.

Computers represent one clear example of a technology that has affected user education. The proliferation of personal computers is documented by the industry itself [34-36]. Health professionals are using computers for literature searching, diagnosis, patient care, research, teaching, continuing education, communicating with colleagues, and other applications. The National Library of Medicine (NLM) promotes its user-friendly searching software program, GRATEFUL MED, directly to health professionals and through libraries. LOANSOME DOC, another NLM product, enables researchers and clinicians to connect to a library's document delivery service and obtain full copies of articles without visiting the library. Commercial vendors have produced telecommunications software, file management programs, computer-assisted instruction, and electronic versions of indexes, textbooks, and journals.

As these products have grown in sophistication, health professionals using them have needed greater understanding of computers, e.g., operating systems, file transfer protocols, and database management, as well as greater understanding of specific library applications. Many of these people have come to librarians for help. The National Library of Medicine, the Medical Library Association, commercial vendors, and individual libraries have targeted clinicians and researchers as end users who need to be taught how to help themselves to information. Anyone in a profession such as medicine, which has a rapidly growing knowledge base, can benefit from knowing how to use electronic databases and computer-assisted instruction.

Why should librarians be teaching the skills required by these computer applications? Because librarians understand record structures, keywords, and the concepts of filing and searching. They know journals and the vagaries of publishing. They know about references and citations. They are in an ideal position to transfer this knowledge to users in an automated environment because they have been searching for years. Long before most people had seen a personal computer, librarians had been sending computerized search requests on punched cards by mail to the National Library of Medicine and taking portable dumb terminals to clinics and labs to perform MEDLINE searches.

There are other reasons for librarians to step onto center stage in the theater of information education:

- Librarians have a generalist's perspective of "the big picture" of information access, management, and use.
- Some users lack alternative access to this type of instruction.
- The neutral turf of the library makes it politically desirable.
- The availability of library classes outside regular curriculum hours can meet users' needs.
- The image of the librarian as confident, helpful, and efficient is enhanced.
- Contact with library users in a different context provides opportunities to learn about other information-related needs.
- A visible and crucial contribution is made to the mission of the parent institution.

In academic settings, everyone benefits from having library educational programs included in the curriculum. Faculty can suggest topics for library assignments that will help students in their classes, librarians will know that the examples suggested are pertinent to students' courses of study, and students will see the relevance of the library instruction.

Librarians have wondered whether they are doing away with their own jobs by teaching users to be self-sufficient; others have pointed out that their role has expanded, since they have become the codesigners and teachers of sophisticated computerized information systems [37-42]. Librarians have taught users the skills needed to become computer literate at a time when users have wanted to exploit the new information systems. Some librarians have been more enthusiastic about encouraging this activity than others. The library literature and presentations at professional meetings over the past decade have reflected the gradual acceptance of training end users as a standard part of library operations [43-49]. Librarians in user education should be teaching whatever skills are needed to retrieve information from the many formats in which it is found, whether from printed pages or electronic sources. Educated users are better able to describe their needs and to know when to rely on librarians for more complex information seeking.

Comments on This Volume

This volume essentially addresses the who, what, when, where, and why of educating users. Abigail Hubbard's chapter, The Context and Ethics of Teaching, includes an excellent discussion of ethics, which are a fundamental consideration in decisions about budgets, audiences, content, and methods of teaching. Her chapter, Teaching and Learning, reaches into the realm of educational theory; it goes beyond *how* to help the reader grasp *why*. This understanding will enable librarians to conduct educational programs in a more effective manner. The current thinking summarized in this chapter can assist library staff in making decisions about design and execution of programs with more knowledge and confidence.

Melanie Wilson and Mary Joan Tooey describe the formats and types of materials used in health sciences library education programs. There are many variations possible, so the authors have limited themselves to the primary ones in use. Abigail Hubbard contributed to the discussions in this chapter of print and nonprint educational materials. As stated here and in Chapter 2: Teaching and Learning, the format and content of instruction take shape from assessing users' needs and documenting realistic goals and objectives.

Providing educational services is expensive in terms of money, time, and new staff expertise. The chapter by Elizabeth Wood, Administration of Educational Services, brings to the reader's attention many aspects of managing educational services, with an emphasis on marketing and staff development. The economics and fees section of this chapter was enhanced with contributions from Abigail Hubbard. Wood also includes a separate section on microcomputer labs and learning centers that covers points notable for teaching. Descriptions of hardware and related subjects are covered in Volume 1 of this series, *Reference and Information Services in Health Sciences Libraries.*

Karla Hahn, Nadia Martin, and Diane Schwartz have synthesized much of what is known about effective evaluation of educational programs. The emphasis is on the utility of the data collected in this process, i.e., how will the information be used? Data collection for its own sake is wasteful and annoying to users and library staff. Readers will avoid such situations if they heed the recommendations of these authors. Their chapter, Evaluation and Future Trends, also summarizes what can be expected to affect educational services in the near future.

In selecting the authors for this volume, a concerted effort was made to include those with hospital or other nonacademic library experience. This search was only partially successful. However, each chapter, and the volume as a whole, was reviewed by both academic and nonacademic librarians. It is hoped that in future editions, librarians from nonacademic settings will step forward as authors. Educational services in hospitals will also be addressed in the second edition of *Hospital Library Management* [50].

A Long-Term View

Educating users to obtain, manage, and evaluate information is truly the domain of librarians. Library staff have an opportunity to develop a strong partnership with health care professionals. The successful creation and marketing of educational services to health care professionals provides librarians with an opportunity to be primary innovators in reshaping professional values concerning how information is acquired, organized, and used [51].

Educational services can be the vehicle to strengthen the library as a strategic player in the health care environment and increase the value of librarians and libraries. This is an extremely important consideration in a time of contracting budgets and downsizing in hospitals, academia, and the public sector. Educational services librarians can have a major impact in redefining the role of libraries in the health care environment.

For the long-term, all library staff can have a vital role in removing the barriers between users and the knowledge and information they seek [52]. Becoming involved in the creation, design, or improvement of systems for information access, management, and use is a critical mission. The future should see no need for a volume on educational services in health sciences libraries if library staff create truly user-friendly systems. This is a challenge for those with vision.

Francesca Allegri
Champaign, Illinois

Acknowledgements

The editor would like to thank the following individuals for their valuable help: Alison Bunting, Editor-in-Chief, for her patient guidance and suggestions. Abigail Hubbard and Elizabeth H. Wood, for their contributions to this Introduction. Sandra L. Wolf for finding the answers to numerous questions during the editing of this volume. She works at the Library and Information Science Library at the University of Illinois at Urbana-Champaign.

References

1. Bandy M. Health information for patients and consumers. In: Holst R, ed. Hospital library management. 2d ed. Metuchen, NJ: Medical Library Association and Scarecrow Press. In preparation.

2. Zachert MJK. Educational services in special libraries: planning and administration. Chicago: Medical Library Association, 1990.

3. Roberts AF, Blandy SG. Library instruction for librarians. 2d rev. ed. Englewood, CO: Libraries Unlimited, 1989.

4. Brottman M, Loe M, eds. The LIRT library instruction handbook. Englewood, CO: Libraries Unlimited, 1990.

5. Dusenbury C, ed. Sourcebook of bibliographic instruction. Chicago: Association of College and Research Libraries, 1993.

6. Wilson LA. Instruction as a reference service. In: Bopp RE, Smith LC, eds. Reference and information services: an introduction. Englewood, CO: Libraries Unlimited, 1991:126-30.

7. Roberts, op. cit., 1-8.

8. Rankin JA, Sayre JW. The educational role of health sciences librarians. Libr Trends 1993 Summer;42(1):45-61.

9. Collins B et al. Introducing computer literacy skills for physicians. Med Ref Serv Q 1992 Winter;11(4):1-9.

10. Frasca MA, Dorsch JL, Aldag JC, Christiansen RG. A multidisciplinary approach to information management and critical appraisal instruction: a controlled study. Bull Med Libr Assoc 1992 Jan;80(1):23-8.

11. Levy SR, Hinegardner PG. Teaching Pro-Cite: classroom instruction and consultations. Med Ref Serv Q 1992 Spring;11(1): 31-7.

12. Moore M. Battling the biomedical information explosion: a plan for implementing a quality filtered database. Med Ref Serv Q 1989 Spring;8(1):13-9.

13. Minchow RL, Pudlock K, Lucas B, Clancy S. Breaking new ground in curriculum integrated instruction. Med Ref Serv Q 1993 Summer;12(2):1-18.

14. Moore M, Schaik JV, Montgomery CL. Physician retraining, lifelong learning, and the library. Bull Med Libr Assoc 1992 Oct;80(4):374-6.

15. Manning PR et al. A method of self-directed learning in continuing medical education with implications for recertification. Ann Intern Med 1987 Dec;107(6):909-13.

16. Arp L. Information literacy or bibliographic instruction: semantics or philosophy? RQ 1990 Fall;30(1):46-9.

17. Breivik PS. Information literacy. Bull Med Libr Assoc 1991 Apr;79(2):226-9.

18. Presidential Committee on Information Literacy. American Library Association. Final Report. Chicago: American Library Association, 1989.

19. Moore M. Innovation and education: unlimited potential for the teaching library. Bull Med Libr Assoc 1989 Jan;77(1):26-32.

20. Arndt KA. Information excess in medicine. Overview, relevance to dermatology, and strategies for coping. Arch Dermatol 1992 Sep;128(9):1249-56.

21. Rudd MJ, Rudd J. The impact of the information explosion on library users: overload or opportunity? J Acad Libr 1986 Nov;12(5):304-7.

22. Cleveland H. The knowledge executive: leadership in an information society. New York: Truman Talley Books, E.P. Dutton, 1985.

23. Lock SP. The future of biomedical communication; a symposium: I. Perspective from the editor of the British Medical Journal.Bull Med Libr Assoc 1992 Apr;80(2):107-9.

24. Love E. Scholarly publishing. Bull Med Libr Assoc 1991 Oct;79(4):408-9.

25. King DN. Creating educational programs in libraries: Part 2: Feasibility. Med Ref Serv Q 1987 Winter;6(4):69-77.

26. Wesley TL. Instructional program design: a re-examination in light of new OPAC demands. Technicalities 1991 Mar;11(3):9-11.

27. King DN. Creating educational programs in libraries: introduction and Part 1: Training and education. Med Ref Serv Q 1987 Fall;6(3):83-90.

28. Hackleman KT, Bischoff FA, eds. Symposium: the evolving role of the health sciences library in continuing education. Bull Med Libr Assoc 1990 Apr;78(2):154-87.

29. Pizer IH. Education—new directions, new constituents. Bull Med Libr Assoc 1989 Oct;77(4):387-8.

30. Darling L, Bishop D, Colaianni LA, eds. Handbook of medical library practice. 4th ed. Chicago: Medical Library Association, 1982-1988.

31. Florance V, Matheson NW. The health sciences librarian as knowledge worker. Libr Trends 1993 Summer;42(1):196-219.

32. Roderer NK. Dissemination of medical information: organizational and technological issues in health sciences libraries. Libr Trends 1993 Summer;42(1):108-26.

33. Messerle J. The changing continuing education role of health sciences libraries. Bull Med Libr Assoc 1990 Apr;78(2):180-7.

34. Arnst C. PC makers head for 'SoHo': 'small-office, home-office' packages are where the growth is. Bus Week 1992 Sep 28;(no. 3285):125-6.

35. O'Malley C. High-tech tools for the home office. Pop Sci 1991 May;238(5):87-90,92,116.

36. O'Malley C. The well-connected home office. Pop Sci 1992 Oct;241(4):90,93.

37. Ojala M. End user searching and its implications for librarians. Spec Libr 1985 Spring;76(2):93-9.

38. Hannigan GG, Brown JF. Managing public access microcomputers in health sciences libraries. Chicago: Medical Library Association, 1990.

39. McCorkel J, Cook V. Computer-assisted instruction: a library service for the community teaching hospital. Bull Med Libr Assoc 1986 Apr;74(2):115-20.

40. Lunin LF, Ball MJ. Perspectives on...information science and health informatics education. J Am Soc Info Sci 1989 Sep;40(5):364-77.

41. Shedlock J. Who's responsible for teaching information management? Med Ref Serv Q 1986 Summer;5(2):77-80.

42. Wood EH. Teaching computer literacy: helping patrons to help themselves. Med Ref Serv Q 1988;7(3):45-57.

43. Auster E, ed. The online searcher. New York: Neal-Schuman, 1990.

44. Glitz B. The role of medical libraries in end-user searching: teaching the MEDLINE database to health care professionals. Sci Tech Libr 1989 Fall;10(1):47-54.

45. Hubbard A, Wilson B. An integrated information management education program...defining a new role for librarians in helping end-users. Online 1986 Mar;10(2):15-23.

46. Hubbard A. Training trainers. Med Ref Serv Q 1988;7(2):63-7.

47. Sollenberger J, Nesbit K. Searching and finding: end user training in the health sciences. Bookmark 1987 Fall;46(1):51-4.

48. Wannarka MB. A training program for the end user in the academic health sciences center. Med Ref Serv Q 1986 Summer;5(2): 95-101.

49. Welborn V, Kuehn JJ. End-user programs in medical school libraries: a survey. Bull Med Libr Assoc 1988 Apr;76(2):137-40.

50. Doyle JD, Wellik KE. Information and educational services. In: Holst R, ed. Hospital library management. 2d ed. Metuchen, NJ: Medical Library Association and Scarecrow Press. In preparation.

51. Urban GL, Hauser JR. Design and marketing of new products. Englewood Cliffs, NJ: Prentice-Hall, 1980.

52. Gorman M. Send for a child of four! or creating the BI-less academic library. Libr Trends 1991 Winter;39(3):354-62.

The Context and Ethics of Teaching

Abigail Hubbard

The Context of Teaching

Two contemporary issues related to teaching underlie the responsibilities of the instructor and learner:

1. People are most comfortable with certainty and predictability—that includes having structure in the way they learn new things. Unfortunately, the need to keep pace with the explosive growth of knowledge renders the notion of predictable structure in learning obsolete.

2. Traditionally, libraries have not been proactive and primary providers of education. The role of libraries in education has been defined externally by library users.

Those who assume the role of teacher are responsible for anticipating the needs of students and creating a learning environment that provides them with the structure to make sense of the vast amounts of information available. Teachers need to create order in the midst of perceived chaos.

The degree of complexity that now exists in the process of information seeking is expressed most elegantly by Briggs and Peat in their book, *Turbulent Mirror,* in which they describe chaos as disorder in a system [1]. Briggs and Peat reveal that in the ancient world, chaos was assumed and accounted for, thus change was not threatening. The development of modern scientific laws has created an illusion of order that allows a false security to develop about the predictability of change. The result is discomfort with change. Finding a means to recapture the comfort level the ancients had with chaos and uncertainty would enable people to make the most of opportunities.

Teachers have the means to reestablish comfort with chaos. They can provide learners with a sense of security and continuity by displaying teaching as a part of an instructional system. That system is designed to predict learning needs and to accommodate the expansion of knowledge. By defining teaching as part of an instructional system, learning can become a part of daily work life. The emphasis of instruction shifts from meeting immediate training needs to allowing learners to take more responsibility for their own intellectual growth.

This approach is a dramatic departure from the way in which instruction is normally perceived. Teaching is seen as a solution to an immediate problem. For example, common responses to a reference desk inundated with students completing a class assignment is to attempt to provide point-of-use instruction for each student or to arrange a class to deal with that particular assignment. Integrating information-seeking skills in the core courses of a curriculum or in courses in which the students receive their research assignments are far more effective responses.

Ethical Considerations

Any complex human interaction, including that which occurs between librarian educators and learners, demands scrutiny from an ethical perspective. This scrutiny assures that basic rights are not violated and that an appropriate and professional working environment is maintained. What follows is an ethical model to guide decisions of this nature.

One might argue that librarians are not confronted with issues grave enough to require a complex model to help them determine appropriate consequences. That is not the case, particularly in the health care environment [2]. Given that there are finite resources, decisions are constantly made in which there are clear winners and equally identifiable losers. Library managers must be capable of making sound decisions about the level of funding for educational endeavors. The staff charged with providing such services must also make allocation decisions that affect program planning and, therefore, distribution of services.

Many models have been developed in other disciplines, such as medicine, business, and law, to describe the boundaries of ethical behavior and to guide the formulation of ethical decisions. The dominant models are derived from Western philosophy [3]. Examining these models will help educational services librarians make sound judgments concerning the ethical results of their work.

Ethical behavior is described primarily using three criteria: *utilitarianism, rights,* and *justice.* A *utilitarian* perspective insures the most favorable result possible for the greatest number of individuals. From the utilitarian perspective, the welfare of the majority is protected at the expense of minority viewpoints. A dilemma emerges when values and perspectives are different between subgroups and coalitions; identifying the correct majority is a problem. An example in the library setting is deciding which groups will be given priority for educational services. To defer to physician requests at the expense of student needs is an example of this kind of judgment. Perhaps students had inadequate advocacy while their educational needs were more compelling than those of the physician group.

The *rights* perspective focuses on individual rights, such as the rights of free speech, free consent, privacy, freedom of conscience, and due process. From a rights perspective, the individual enjoys protection and personal entitlements at the expense of other individuals or groups. For example, a librarian may believe he or she has a right to refuse instructional services to a group that opposes his or her viewpoint on abortion. The question is whether the right to freedom of conscience protects the librarian. Guarding individual rights is independent of results, which can lead to diminished productivity and efficiency. A rights perspective can be disruptive if it leads to extremely individualistic behavior.

The *justice* perspective focuses on equitable treatment, fairness in the interpretation of rules and policies, and remuneration for violation of a person's rights. This particular perspective is strongly egalitarian and democratic. In a library setting, there may be a perception that the same level of educational services should be provided for every user group. This interpretation is incorrect because fairness does not mean sameness; it simply means fair judgments will be made concerning treatment of individuals. Because of misinterpretation, there is a strong possibility that individual rights will be violated in favor of perceived equity.

For a decision to be unequivocally ethical, none of these three criteria (utilitarianism, rights, or justice) can be violated. Such an occurrence is rare. Inevitably, the protection of the rights of the majority will violate the individual rights of a few, and application of justice criteria frequently will violate individual rights. Conversely, protection of individual rights frequently will violate both utilitarian and justice criteria. Judgment is always required in determining whether behavior is ethical.

To resolve this dilemma, the concept of testing for overwhelming effects was formulated. One such situation is known as double effect, in which a decision will lead to two outcomes, one good and one bad. The choice is acceptable if the magnitude of good effect is significant enough to outweigh the bad effect.

As ethics become more ambiguous, the quality of decisions becomes more important. Careful consideration is needed. When standards of conduct, product quality, or service quality become unclear, sanctions are greater. The stakes are higher.

All decisions will reflect the dominant values present in a system and be moderated by minority values. An example in the library is whether service priorities are customer driven or for the convenience of library staff. Maintaining an appropriate perspective about why the library exists, i.e., for users, is important. Another serious question to ask is: Are values primarily defined by library staff or are they defined externally? Librarians can and should define and reinforce values that explicitly favor the library's user group. Otherwise, a forceful external coalition may impose its values on the library. Librarians must define the standards for their conduct and for the quality of their services while accommodating the value system(s) of their user population.

References

1. Briggs J, Peat FD. Turbulent mirror: an illustrated guide to chaos theory and the science of wholeness. New York: Harper & Row, 1989.

2. Gray SA, Widzinski LJ. Information technology in the health sciences library: an ethical perspective. Med Ref Serv Q 1993 Summer;12(2):45-55.

3. Cavanagh GF, Mogerg DJ, Velasquez M. The ethics of organizational politics. Acad Manage Rev 1981 Jul;6(3):363-74.

2

Teaching and Learning

Abigail Hubbard

The "sink or swim" method of learning to propel oneself through the water is frightening at best and fatal at worst. Learning to teach does not have to be that stressful. By studying the theoretical underpinnings of teaching and learning, the reader can

- Intelligently observe the teaching practices of others.
- Improve one's own effectiveness.
- Conserve energy and resources.
- Feel more comfortable in a teaching role.

This chapter provides a framework for the rest of this volume. The theory presented here underlies the activities, administration, and evaluation of educational services.

The swimming analogy also underscores the importance of the issues presented in this chapter. One can squander a great deal of energy doing the dog paddle, or one can glide through the water with an efficient and effortless-looking crawl stroke. Library staff will save time and money if the points discussed here are taken to heart. They help answer questions such as what type of instruction is best suited to a particular audience, how much information should be presented, and what kinds of activities would reinforce learning.

This chapter begins by explaining why teaching is a social contract and why that concept is useful, followed by a discussion of the learner and the teacher. Next, the instructional systems-design process is described, including delivery systems and learning theory. Finally, the process of teaching is outlined.

Teaching as a Social Contract

Teaching is a social contract between a teacher and a learner. Specific responsibilities and obligations must be honored by both parties in order for the terms of the contract to be fulfilled. Social contracts are usually ambiguous and ill-defined; the relationship between the teacher and the learner needs to be clarified. The responsibilities and obligations of both parties will be explored in the following pages.

The Learner

One of the luxuries of teaching in a health sciences library environment is that the students are adults. Adult learners exhibit very distinct characteristics that make teaching challenging yet rewarding. Knowles categorizes these characteristics as *behavioral, emotional,* or *cognitive* [1].

Behavioral characteristics of adults include the following:

- Adults express different motives for pursuing education than younger students. Adult motives focus on improvement of professional or economic status and self-actualization.
- Many adults exhibit group behaviors inconsistent with what is perceived to be the norm in a classroom. Adults expect a collegial atmosphere and an opportunity to interact freely with both the teacher and fellow learners. For example, adults who collaborate in a research laboratory may be accustomed to spontaneous, spirited discussion and debate. These adults are likely to exhibit similar behavior in a classroom setting. A teacher who is expecting passive students may be unprepared to handle the challenges of this kind of situation.
- Adults typically respond to reinforcements that have meaning in their work environment. With students in medical, nursing, or other health care curricula, it is useful and appropriate to adopt the grading system used by their schools. However, such rewards are ineffective with practicing health care professionals, e.g., grades are generally of no consequence. The opportunity to learn is important, and grades should only be used when they fit the context of the learner.
- Adults normally work and live in an environment where it is expected that they will appear to be in control. Because of this expectation, adults

tend to display restricted emotional responses in a traditional learning environment.

- Many adults have set habits and have developed strong biases and preconceptions. These behavioral tendencies and preferred beliefs may restrict an adult's willingness to try new methods of learning.
- Adults bring to learning a rich history of personal experiences. From this basis of experience, adults will seek parallels to what they are currently learning, and this will shape their responses. Adults will seek to fit new knowledge into their established patterns.

Emotional characteristics of adults include the following:

- Many adults have a fear of falling behind and being replaced. They may feel pressure to remain current so that they can retain their positions in an increasingly competitive environment.
- Adults seek social interaction with their peers through educational experiences.
- Adults may be very preoccupied with concerns outside a given learning situation, causing their attention to waver or fade.
- Adults are frequently intimidated by change.
- Many adults are uncomfortable in the student role.
- Adults are very concerned about how they invest their time.
- Adults are sometimes bewildered by their options, but fearful of expressing their discomfort.
- Life experiences have led most adults to filter influences (stimuli) selectively.
- Adults generally have very strong feelings about learning situations and expected results.
- Adults have very tangible things to lose and sometimes fear the loss of those things.
- A primary strength and limitation of adults as learners is their mature emotional framework of values, attitudes, and commonly expressed behaviors.

Cognitive characteristics of adults include the following:

- Adults tend to reject new information that does not fit their personal belief system. This process is known as selective retention.

- Adults develop associations with known stimuli that assist or hinder learning. For example, adults may react positively to a teacher's critique during a classroom practice session because previous feedback, or knowledge of results, helped them learn. Conversely, if adults' questions were perceived by others as unsophisticated or inappropriate they may not voice them because of potential embarrassment.
- Adults bring to new learning experiences a well-developed learning style and an ability to express their own preferences.
- Adults quickly identify the relevance or irrelevance of new information and experiences. New relevant knowledge is rapidly accepted and assimilated into their repertoires.
- Adults learn faster and retain far more when they perceive a direct relationship between new information and present needs.

The value of understanding the behavioral, emotional, and cognitive needs of individuals is unquestioned, but it does not provide a complete profile of adults as learners. There are some other factors that define the relationship between the librarian as teacher and the health care professional as student. Understanding these factors will result in a more satisfying educational experience for both.

Factors in the Teacher-Learner Relationship

Self-Selection

Most participants in library educational programs choose to attend because they find the content relevant to their professional work. They discern a benefit from investing their time in their own continuing education. The librarian educator needs to expend energy in the instructional design process to identify precisely what the health care professional values in an educational experience.

Collegial Status

Many who assume the role of student in library educational programs are faculty, researchers, or health care professionals. These are the librarian's professional peers. This has implications for the instructional design of the learning experience, the style of teaching selected, and the selection and arrangement of the physical facilities in which instruction is to take place.

Authority Figure Status

Because most of the students are professionals, they are authority figures in their own right. The traditional teacher-student role positions the teacher in the authority role and the student in a submissive role. Adult learners do not respond well in that situation. Adults are likely to feel negative about previous unsuccessful learning experiences. They may express hostility and resentment overtly or nonverbally during the course of instruction. This behavior is disruptive to the class and influences the choice of teaching style.

Expertise

All participants in a class bring expertise unique to their chosen specialty. While they may be an expert in their field, rarely are they an expert in information management. The collective wisdom and intelligence of the participants in the room may be intimidating to some instructors. Maintaining perspective on one's own skill and value will help the instructor retain the self-confidence needed to be successful. Participants are there because they have a need to learn what is being offered.

Respect

Recognizing the importance of class participants' roles in delivering health care, and according them the respect they presume, will usually result in a more productive instructional environment.

Instructional librarians will recognize in themselves the same set of characteristics described here, for they are adult learners, also. Being able to identify with the learner enables the instructor to create a successful learning experience. What distinguishes the adult learner from the instructor is role definition. Articulating roles and acknowledging mutual and individual strengths allows learners to accept their function without negative peer judgment or loss of self-esteem. Understanding this form of social exchange helps the instructor accommodate students' needs, be they emotional, behavioral, or cognitive.

The Teacher

There is intense debate about whether teaching is an art or a science. Interesting essays and books abound [2-4]. A common theme is the emotive response that teaching triggers for many people. These supporters argue that teaching is an art that cannot be defined, that it comes from the heart, and that some people are born teachers.

Teaching can be personally rewarding and does have an emotive quality about it, but teaching can be learned. This is important and comforting to know, because adult learners are very demanding and typically require that their teachers be technically competent individuals. Content orientation and expertise are extremely important in a classroom. There is a compelling argument to be made that the experts should learn to be teachers, rather than assume that an expert teacher can teach anything [5]. An interesting parallel exists in the workplace; acceptance of managers hinges on technical competence [6].

Taking librarian experts and placing them in a classroom can make them very uncomfortable. Novice teachers should be given a chance to learn and achieve a reasonable comfort level prior to planning and teaching their first class. Methods should be in place to provide new teachers with help and feedback. These steps help integrate instructors into the program. Experts who have become excellent teachers seem to agree that reading about teaching, observing others, practice, and feedback were the most useful in learning to teach. (For more information on training and development of teachers, see Chapter 4.)

Instructional Systems-Design Process

When an educational or training deficiency is identified, the following steps need to be taken:

- Assess the need from the perspective of the target audience.
- Design appropriate instruction.
- Implement the instruction.
- Evaluate its effectiveness.

This process is more complex than responding to a request for microcomputer training with a prefabricated three-hour workshop. Instructional design using a systems perspective assumes several things. The most important assumption is that instructional design is a process, not a product. Litzinger provides an overview of the process [7]. Carson and Curtis provide a detailed description of instructional design as it relates to bibliographic instruction [8-10].

It is unrealistic to believe that all health sciences librarians will be able to undertake instructional systems design as described here. If financial, staffing, or other constraints make needs assessment or design of instruction impossible, the systems-design process can be adjusted. For example, commercially produced materials or those created at other libraries can be used if they have been examined for suitability to the audience and the stated objectives. In some settings, librarians may have detailed knowledge of their users, which would permit a less formal needs assessment process. However, librarians should also work to improve support for educational services. One way to do this is to capitalize on the value to users of successful programs. A catch-22 exists here; sacrifices are needed to competently fulfill the library's educational mission. In the meantime, the content provided in the following sections is presented as a goal.

Educators must recognize that instructional systems design exploits all the components of organizational systems, including:

- Appropriate use of inputs.
- Determination of optimal processes.
- Development of outputs.
- Sensitivity to feedback from all facets of the environment.

The importance of feedback cannot be overemphasized. Feedback provides an opportunity to keep the system thriving. The obligation of health care professionals to possess information-seeking skills makes cutting-edge instruction mandatory.

To successfully use the instructional systems-design process, there are several issues that require greater attention.

Target Audience Analysis

The participants' general characteristics need to be analyzed from two perspectives: individual and organizational. This analysis gives the instructor an understanding of what the potential students already know, so that instruction is planned at an appropriate level. The analysis also provides some clues about how to present new information to the learners. Some of the information to be gathered about participants includes the following:

- What are the participants' goals?
- Why do they value the proposed instruction?
- What is the academic background of the participants?
- What organizations or departments are represented?

- What is the status of the participants within their organization?
- What is the background of these participants?
- How will they be using the information presented in the seminar, workshop, or class?
- What experiences have the participants had relative to the subject matter of the seminar, workshop, or class?
- What kind of time constraints are in effect for participants?
- How do participants view the library and the librarian's role?

When the answers to these questions are examined, it will be found that some groups are conveniently homogeneous, while others are heterogeneous in their composition. Homogeneity allows focused instruction; heterogeneity requires difficult decisions on the part of the instructor to determine the emphasis and process of the instruction.

For example, if some of the participants have a great deal of experience with the content of the course but the remainder have little or none, the instructor must decide how complex the content will be. This decision will favor either the experienced or inexperienced participants. If the instruction is targeted to the lowest common denominator in the group, the majority of the participants may be bored or irritated. If instruction is focused at the high end of participants' knowledge level, many will leave the instructional experience frustrated, lost, or confused.

Changing the composition of the group may be needed. One way to do this is to subdivide the group by experience level. In the case of educational offerings open to anyone, advertising should explicitly state the skills and knowledge level needed by attendees. (For other ideas and examples of target audience analysis, see the section on marketing in Chapter 4.)

An additional target audience issue is reward structures. Because educational services librarians are working predominantly with adult learners, the desired rewards are different from those associated with students in a more traditional educational environment. For adults, acquired knowledge and confidence is usually the greatest reward [11].

The basic criteria for any reward is that it must be valued by the recipient. Offering any additional rewards to participants must follow this principle [12]. As noted earlier in discussing behavioral characteristics of adults, traditional grades are totally inappropriate. Grades are an artifact of a structured educational system that uses them both as rewards and sanctions. Adult learners are not seeking sanctions, they are seeking knowledge. The acquisition of relevant, immediately useful information is highly valued. In addition, careful, considered feedback is important to an adult learner.

Needs Assessment

A needs assessment is conducted for the sole purpose of identifying discrepancies between current performance or knowledge levels and expected performance or knowledge levels. As mentioned earlier, this step can be modified according to a particular library's constraints. Investing the time and resources required to conduct a needs assessment pays off in many ways:

- It identifies real, rather than perceived, instructional needs.
- It demonstrates a commitment to planning.
- It ensures effective use of resources by investing in the most critical instructional needs.

As with any systematic study, attention to the details of data collection will have a profound effect on the quality of the needs assessment. Useful information must be collected and analyzed, including who the target audience is, what is important to them, how they use information, and other characteristics.

If time and resources for conducting the needs assessment are scarce, it may make sense to employ ethnographic or qualitative methodologies for analysis. Ethnographic methods involve in-depth study and depiction of a specific population using naturalistic, participant-observer methods [13].

Focus groups and long interview techniques help assess target audience values. Focus groups provide an opportunity for peers to engage in open discussions in a nonthreatening environment. These discussions are observed by a facilitator who can seek clarification and elaboration of issues that are raised. The focus group can be followed by in-depth interviews with selected members of the target audience who express concerns representative of the larger group.

Surveys may be an appropriate method of collecting information from a large number of users. An effective survey instrument can be constructed by interviewing or using focus groups with a sample of the proposed participants. Data collected with the survey instruments can be analyzed by common statistical methods.

Educational services librarians need to remember that proactive education as a library service is a relatively new idea for users to embrace. As such, librarians need to invoke models for dissemination of innovation such as co-opting innovators and early adopters to sell library educational services. Actively involving members of the target audience in the data collection process helps participants more fully understand and appreciate library educational services. Focus groups and long interviews help create cultural bonds through shared values. These bonds motivate innovators and early adopters to support new ideas.

Goals and Objectives

Once specific education or training needs have been identified, goals and objectives must be written to address these needs. An instructional goal should explicitly describe expected results of the instruction, whether the results are in the cognitive, affective, or psychomotor domains of learning. Goals usually focus on the ideal, rather than the satisfactory or suboptimal [14].

Objectives help teachers plan the instructional experience and should be specific, measurable, realistic, achievable, and related to goal attainment. Awareness of objectives, from the start, by both teacher and learner helps maintain a focus and assures that the instruction is meeting its stated purpose. Model statements of objectives are described in the literature [15-16].

A taxonomy, or classification, of instructional objectives is an additional aid to teachers. It establishes a common terminology for design and evaluation of education. A taxonomy of objectives also suggests other instructional results that the teacher may not have considered. The most widely cited taxonomies of educational objectives are those developed by Bloom [17-18]. Harrow developed a third taxonomy [19]. These classifications outline objectives for the cognitive, affective, and psychomotor domains on a continuum of complexity.

The type of instructional delivery system, e.g., lecture, discussion, or simulation, that is selected by an instructor has a limiting effect on the level of objective that can be achieved. For example, if an instructor chooses to deliver content using a lecture, learning success theoretically can be achieved only at the lowest levels of Bloom's taxonomy: knowledge and comprehension. To achieve application, analysis, synthesis, or evaluation would require, at a minimum, that group discussion take place to allow for reinforcement of values and more complete knowledge acquisition.

Instructors need to understand the impact that their delivery system has on achieving their objectives. If the choice of delivery systems is limited, it may be necessary to rewrite objectives.

Content Analysis

When goals and objectives have been defined, it is time to determine appropriate content for the instruction. Content analysis requires a subject matter expert (SME). If the person responsible for designing the instruction is not an expert on the topic identified, a team consisting of the instructional designer and the subject expert or experts will be needed. For example, the reference librarian designing an online catalog session would find it useful to team up with a member of the cataloging department. The size of the team depends on the complexity of the content.

Organizing the content of the instruction in a manner appropriate for the target audience is the responsibility of the instructional designer, with the guidance of the SME. To assure accuracy, the SME must sign off on the content outline before the instruction is produced and delivered. Content analysis is a time-consuming process. There is a strong need to communicate clearly and accurately to a target audience that, in all likelihood, has had little prior instruction related to libraries or information management.

Hierarchy of Learning

An important caveat must be expressed when the librarian designing the instruction is also the content expert. It is very difficult for an expert to communicate at an appropriate level to a novice or intermediate-level learner. To understand why this is so, it is useful to examine a hierarchy of learning.

Level 1: Unconsciously Incompetent

At this level, learners are too naive about the subject matter to be aware of their deficiencies or to understand what learning needs to take place.

> **Example:** A lab technician is aware that microcomputers exist, but is not aware of how or why they might be useful in her environment.

Level 2: Consciously Incompetent

Learners are now aware of their deficiencies and of what needs to be learned.

> **Example:** The lab technician is now aware of precisely how the use of a microcomputer will make her job more efficient, but has no knowledge about how to use the computer.

Level 3: Consciously Competent

At this level, learners have mastered the information necessary to perform at prescribed levels, but are very aware of the processes or skills they are using to complete the task.

Example: Now the lab technician has acquired training on how to use a microcomputer and how to apply it to analyze lab data. The technician can perform specific tests, and very carefully and conscientiously thinks about each keystroke and command as she uses the computer.

Level 4: Unconsciously Competent

Learners have now mastered the information or skill and have had adequate practice and feedback to perform without consciously thinking about what steps to follow or what processes to invoke to complete tasks.

Example: The lab technician has been using a microcomputer to assist her with routine analyses for several months. The processes and steps for using the computer have become second nature, and she no longer thinks about which keys must be hit to invoke common commands. The process has become intuitive [20].

An instructional designer who is also a content expert is quite likely operating at Level 4, or unconsciously competent. It is very difficult to back up to the level of consciously competent to insure that all essential information is conveyed to a novice learner. Another content person can help review the outline before completing the instructional design. A novice in the subject area may see gaps more easily.

Delivery Systems

Once the content outline has been completed, a decision must be made concerning the appropriate method of instruction (the delivery system). This decision will be based on the target audience, the results of the needs assessment, the goals and objectives, and the content outline. The method of delivery must fit into the standard activity patterns of the target audience. It must also take into account the following factors:

- Learning styles.
- Time constraints.
- Comfort with technology.
- Availability of technology.
- Financial constraints.
- Geographic limitations.

The first of these, learning styles, may be an esoteric concept. Because it is fundamental to choice of delivery systems, the following description is provided for clarification.

Learning Theory

Familiarity with major learning theories can help an instructor understand how students master new concepts and skills. Discussing each learning theory in depth is beyond the scope of this chapter, but it is useful to know that different people approach learning in different ways. Learning styles, factors in the teacher-learner relationship, and characteristics of adult learners are all important in designing and delivering instruction.

Three commonly cited learning theories are *behaviorism, developmental theory,* and *cognitive theory* [21-23]. Skinnerian *behaviorism* introduced the notion of stimulus-response and the importance of reinforcement (feedback). The primary limitation of behaviorism for teaching is that it assumes a passive learner. Behaviorism is also a linear process and does not consider the complexity inherent in learning some knowledge and skills.

Piaget emphasized stages of cognitive *development* and contended that information needs to be presented at a level that is the same as that of the learner. Many of the rules-of-thumb accepted about teaching are based on the precepts of the developmental theory. As a result, teachers attempt to employ a style that is compatible with the age, experience, and level of cognitive development of the learner.

A third approach in describing how humans learn is labeled the *cognitive,* or information-processing, theory. This approach suggests that humans process information in a manner similar to the way that computer functions are described: input (perception), processing, storage, retrieval (of information), and output (appropriate to the situation). The information-processing theory allows for repetition and branching that are learner specific. It is inferred that learning is a complex operation contingent on the cognitive processes of the individual. These processes are moderated by practice, feedback, and experience.

Learning theories have been applied in recognizing how individuals approach learning and what the implications are for an instructor. Various instruments have been used to identify a person's general approach to learning. One of the most commonly used instruments is the Learning Style Instrument (LSI), developed by David Kolb [24]. As with any instrument, this one has detractors, but it illustrates this discussion [25].

Kolb developed an instrument that categorized learning style preferences in one of four ways: concrete experience, abstract conceptualization, active experimentation, and reflective observation [26]. By understanding characteristics of people who prefer each of these learning styles, one can determine teaching methods that usually work, as well as those that do not work, for each learning style. This approach is not only useful for group instruction, but for one-on-one instruction, as well [27].

Concrete Experience

These learners tend to prefer an experiential approach to learning that relies heavily on feelings-based judgments. Although it is not possible to learn without experience of some kind, the type of experiences referred to here are drawn from the learners' work and everyday life [28]. These learners are typically people oriented, more comfortable with peers than authority figures, and inclined to be empathic. Teaching methods that appeal to concrete experience learners include the use of specific examples, feedback, and discussion. Learning by doing is more successful with these individuals than are theoretical approaches.

Abstract Conceptualization

Abstract conceptualizers tend to be analytical and rely heavily on logical thinking and rational evaluation. They are inclined to be oriented more toward things than people. Teaching methods that appeal to abstract conceptualizers use impersonal learning situations with an emphasis on theory and systematic analysis of concepts. These learners do not respond well to unstructured approaches, exercises, or simulations.

Active Experimentation

These learners tend to prefer an active, *doing* orientation to learning that relies heavily on experimentation. They are generally extroverted by nature. Teaching methods that appeal to active experimenters include hands-on projects, group discussions, and homework (exercises they can take away and do on their own). They do not respond well to passive learning techniques such as lectures.

Reflective Observation

Reflective observers tend to have a tentative, impartial, reflective approach to learning. Their orientation is primarily introverted, relying heavily on careful scrutiny in making judgments. Teaching methods that appeal to reflective observers are lectures and methods that allow learning through observation. Less successful teaching approaches include group discussions, exercises, simulations, and role playing.

What do these styles mean when teaching heterogeneous groups of adults with whom the instructor has no previous experience? Of course, a teacher cannot predict individual learning styles with a glance around the room. These descriptions of styles make it clear that people bring to the learning experience strong biases in how they choose to digest new information. An instructor can assume, with most groups, that the entire range of learning styles is represented. By understanding that these biases exist, and are quite strong in some cases, instructors can plan their teaching to create opportunities for diverse learners to feel comfortable and grasp the information presented.

Instructors can also direct learners to alternatives that support independent learning, such as computer-assisted instruction or programmed workbooks. Creative technological developments have provided instructional designers with a wide range of choices in delivery systems. These are discussed in detail in Chapter 3. The most common option is described in the following paragraphs to illustrate how learning styles apply.

Classroom Instruction

Perhaps the most familiar model of instruction is the traditional classroom. Students receive information from an instructor who uses lecture, discussion, small group process, or a combination of these methods. Understanding when to use these alternate methods in the classroom is valuable.

Lectures are effective for the following:

- Introducing new content.
- Orienting students to a new topic.
- Providing directions for subsequent activities.
- Presenting rapidly changing information.

Reflective learners usually enjoy lectures, while active learners tend to get frustrated. A strong, competent delivery is needed for a lecture to be productive for either type of learner. Lecturers should avoid reading notes verbatim, because that leads to artificiality. Listeners may perceive that the instructor is insincere, lacks self-confidence, or lacks mastery of the subject. Instead, the lecturer should use brief notes and allow for spontaneity. The lecturer should also show a personal interest in the topic, use appropriate and comfortable gestures and movements, maintain eye contact, and remain poised and relaxed.

Group discussions are extremely effective when attempting to influence fundamental values or address a controversial topic. Being an effective discussion leader is more difficult than lecturing, because of the dynamic flow of content and the unpredictable interactions among participants. Leading a group discussion requires careful preparation and planning to assure that objectives are met. To that end, discussion leaders commonly make contingency plans that include pertinent content, challenging questions, and summary points. Perhaps the most difficult challenge for a good discussion leader is to remain emotionally disengaged from the deliberations and concentrate on shaping the focus of discussion and providing opportunities for students to participate [29].

Small group process includes the use of problem solving and experiential exercises. Because adults frequently enjoy the social part of the educational experience, group problem solving is particularly effective. Providing a realistic situation, as in a case study, works because adults bring a breadth of knowledge to the learning experience. They can learn from each other in a nonthreatening manner. Experiential exercises might be problematic if the learners anticipate that the situation could be embarrassing or uncomfortable. Understanding the target audience is crucial to planning successful learning experiences.

The role of the instructor is that of facilitator and resource person, rather than active participant. The role of the teacher becomes more passive and the role of the student becomes more active as the instructional method moves from lecture to group discussion to small group process.

Focusing on the needs of the students and matching the delivery system to these needs can be difficult for instructors who have become comfortable with one particular method of instruction. Expanding one's repertoire benefits students. Also, it can make teaching more fun and postpone burnout indefinitely.

Evaluation

Evaluation is a feedback process that is critical for any system to survive or thrive. Specifics of evaluation are discussed in Chapter 5, but a few points need to be stressed here. Evaluation of teaching provides the instructor with information that contributes to improvement in both the teaching process and the instructional design process. For evaluation to be useful, data collection instruments and processes must be fashioned to elicit the information needed. Primary issues are how the information will be used and who will have access to it. These are managerial and ethical questions. The design of the information-gathering process will be different if the information will be used by managers for performance appraisal, salary, and position decisions, as opposed to being used by the instructor and instructional designer to improve learners' performance. (For a discussion of ethics as they relate to instruction, see Chapter 1.)

Data collection needs to be devised to provide students with an opportunity to fairly evaluate discrete aspects of their experience. A student should be able to negatively evaluate one aspect of an educational experience while positively responding to other issues. Therefore, ambiguity should be reduced by careful design of data-collection instruments and processes. Areas to evaluate include content, level of instruction, instructor, and physical environment.

An instructional designer can help critique the design and execution of educational programs. For librarians working in an academic setting, these kinds of resources are frequently available to help faculty improve their teaching skills. Members of professional associations can also help, including members of the National Society for Performance and Instruction and the American Society for Training and Development. (For addresses, see Appendix A.)

The Process of Teaching

Heuristics, or rules-of-thumb, can help teachers by providing guidelines for cultivating new approaches to teaching. Several general issues are identified here, with some suggested heuristics that will help achieve success in teaching.

Organize Content Logically

There are many ways to define, describe, categorize, and organize a body of information. How an instructor chooses to organize the content will have a profound effect on the results.

- Maintain the students' perspective when determining the logic and arrangement of the content. Each profession defines and describes knowledge in a distinct manner. In addition, the context of the new information must be appropriately identified.
- Avoid making incorrect assumptions about the student knowledge base. One risks presenting information from a perspective that is too naive or overly sophisticated.

- Recognize one's own bias in teaching style when organizing content.

Motivate Students

One of the most important motivational tools an instructor has is the ability to link the content of the educational experience to the learner's personal and professional value system.

- Explain why this learning opportunity has relevance and why it is important enough to be allocated personal time, energy, and, in some cases, money.
- Project enthusiasm about teaching and a real interest in the students and the topic.

Identify the Benefits of the Knowledge

Establish one's own credibility as an instructor. Be certain that students understand the instructor's role and expertise, as well as how an instructor can provide something of value to them in exchange for their time and energy.

- Establish a rapport with students. Remember that instructors share the same adult learner characteristics as their students.
- Honestly empathize with student concerns.

Establish the Context for the Content

Help learners explain how and why the information or skills they are seeking fit into their personal work environment.

- Relate the content of the learning experience to the personal and work experiences of the participants, using their own professional language, jargon, and examples to provide greater understanding.
- Suggest alternative approaches to traditional work habits that are made possible as a result of learning new information or skills.

Identify the Structure of the Experience

Ambiguity often makes people uncomfortable. Anything that instructors can do to reduce uncertainty in a learning situation will enhance the ability of participants to focus on the primary agenda rather than their discomfort.

- Provide an explicit agenda for the learning experience.
- Verbally emphasize the important points to be covered.
- Provide a specific timetable that identifies breaks and finish times.

Create a Comfortable Physical Environment

The primary reason for attending to physical surroundings is to eliminate distractions from the primary agenda. If a person is cold, if there is too much noise filtering into the room, or if the instructor cannot be heard, the learner's attention is diverted from learning to these distractions.

- Make certain that temperature, lighting, noise levels, and the physical arrangement of furniture are appropriate for the activities to be conducted.
- Project one's voice so that all can hear clearly, or use a microphone to do so.
- Provide adequate breaks during long classes or seminars.
- Allow participants to choose their own seating.
- Be tolerant of individual needs. In a health care environment, participants may need to leave unexpectedly or keep in close touch with their offices or clinics.

Control Student Attention

Understand that a teacher has the responsibility to provide a stimulating environment for learning. Teachers compete with a number of antecedent conditions characteristic of adult learners. Adult learners bring to the classroom their preoccupation with their work; their attention may wander back to a work problem encountered earlier in the day.

- Open the class or seminar in an unusual manner, providing an interesting mental hook for the participants.
- Use audiovisual aids.
- Plan student participation where appropriate.
- Provide ongoing summaries of cogent points.

Control Student Activities

Adult learners who have made a commitment to invest time and energy in an educational experience usually demand results. Adults also want a comfortable, nonthreatening environment in which to learn. A teacher should prepare adequately to guarantee students the experience they expect.

- Provide written outlines, summaries, and examples to lessen the need for students to take notes. Taking notes robs a student of the opportunity to process and analyze the information just received. Explain the structure and level of detail of the notes, so students can adapt them to their needs.
- Structure activities to allow for instructor intervention or termination. Adults do not appreciate having their time wasted with what they perceive to be irrelevant activities. Be ready and willing to abort exercises that prove ineffective and substitute other relevant activities.

Use Examples and Analogies Whenever Possible

Learners need to be provided with a basis for comparison so they can assimilate information and apply their new knowledge to their experiences [30].

- Use relevant examples from the learner's typical environment.
- Use examples and analogies to provide a point of reference or platform for the introduction of more complex concepts.
- Capitalize on the past experiences of the learners to assist their future learning.

Omit Extraneous Materials

Adult learners generally are focused and demanding in a learning environment. Adults require relevance. Eliminating nonessential information should be accomplished in the instructional design process when identifying the target audience and defining the instructional need.

- Don't let details overshadow important points.
- Allow appropriate time for each individual concept or task.
- Keep in mind the attention span of students. Normally, adults can assimilate only six new major concepts per hour (details can supplement the new concepts). After forty-five minutes, there should be a scheduled break [31].

Integrate Practice and Interaction Where Appropriate

The proactive participation of libraries in education and the notion that health care professionals should be responsible for managing their information needs are both relatively new concepts. Because of this, there is a significant component of user education programs devoted to helping potential learners embrace the value of what libraries offer. The most effective way to transmit and reinforce values is through peer discussion. Interaction among learners should have a high priority.

- Allow discussions and debate of issues among participants, providing guidance and clarification when required.
- Inject activities and discussions into otherwise passive learning experiences.
- Provide hands-on experience to allow the instructor to observe the student and provide feedback needed for skill mastery.

Provide Constant Feedback

Feedback enables adjustment of the primary processes, in this case, teaching. Feedback helps the instructor identify success or failure on the part of both the instructor and the student and make modifications as needed.

- Answer questions at the time they are asked, if possible.
- When the response to a question is, "We will cover that later...," be certain to call attention to the question later in the session, when it is answered. This provides closure for the students and reinforces their confidence in the ability of the instructor to provide a meaningful learning experience.
- Listen and watch for verbal and nonverbal cues that participants are understanding or confused. An instructor can confirm these observations through comments or questions such as, "There seems to be some confusion...." This lets the instructor and students clarify a concept. The instructor should constantly adjust the learning experience, based on such observations and feedback.

Summarize

Summary statements provide students with a framework for the experiences they are about to have or have just completed.

- At the beginning of a class or seminar, provide an overview.
- Provide ongoing summaries of cogent points, linking current issues and ideas to those previously stated.

- Review the progress of the learning experience with students to validate common understandings and reinforce expectations.
- At the conclusion of the learning experience, provide an overview emphasizing the acquisition of practical knowledge. Allow the learners to participate in this summary.

Respond to Challenging Students

To categorize a student as a problem is purely perceptual. One instructor may respond to a student very negatively and label the student's behavior disruptive and inappropriate. Another instructor may perceive the same student to be an intellectually challenging person with a wonderful mind for debate. Aggression is often a response to an emotional issue, and it is inappropriate for an instructor to engage students in that manner.

All instructors encounter challenging students and need to be able to tactfully address the problems they present while allowing the students to save face among their peers. Students who participate in library-sponsored educational opportunities are professional peers as well as library users. Librarians have a relationship with these users that will continue long after the uncomfortable classroom experience.

- Don't offend students or insult their intelligence.
- Offer comments with a positive perspective.
- Don't offer excuses for content, delivery, unforeseen events, the library, or other students.
- Defer irrelevant comments to a meeting after class. Offer to discuss student concerns or topics with them in more depth at a separate meeting. Tactfully remind them of the scope of the current educational experience.
- Acknowledge the students' expertise. In some cases, the students want their personal perspective or expertise validated. Examples of comments an instructor might employ to diffuse an aggressive student include:

"You seem to be quite advanced in this area; your personal knowledge seems to go beyond the scope of this seminar."

"Perhaps an advanced seminar would be more appropriate for you. We can discuss those after class, if you wish."

"You present an interesting perspective. Unfortunately, we don't have time within the scope of this class to explore that issue in depth."

The Opportunities

Any new professional opportunity, such as teaching, should be an experience to relish and immerse oneself in. This notion was elegantly expressed by Gibbs in *Dancing with Your Books: The Zen Way of Studying* [32]. Gibbs advocates that people should accept where they are and what they are doing at the moment and do the best that they can. His advice was targeted at college students who might prefer to be anywhere but a lecture hall, but it applies to any situation. What is called *work* and what is called *play* is a matter of perspective. Teaching can be enormously fun or overwhelmingly stressful. The difference in personal outcome is defined by preparation and commitment.

Teachers are also learners and are not infallible. Every venture into a classroom is an opportunity to learn more and to try new skills. Good lecturers often say that they learn more than their students when they deliver a good lecture. Perhaps the most beneficial advice for anyone who chooses to teach is to approach teaching with the same vigor, enthusiasm, and tenacity as one would any chosen professional role. The more energy invested in learning the tools of the trade, the more enjoyable the experience.

References

1. Knowles MS. The adult learner: a neglected species. 4th ed. Houston: Gulf, 1990.

2. Ericksen SC. The essence of good teaching. San Francisco: Jossey Bass, 1984.

3. Gullette MM, ed. The art and craft of teaching. Cambridge: Harvard University, 1984.

4. Eble KE, ed. Improving teaching styles. San Francisco: Jossey Bass, 1980. (New directions for teaching and learning, no. 1.)

5. Fraher R. Learning a new art: suggestions for beginning teachers. In: Gullette MM, ed. The art and craft of teaching. Cambridge: Harvard University, 1984:116-27.

6. Miller DB. Managing professionals in research and development. San Francisco: Jossey Bass, 1986.

7. Litzinger ME. Instructional design. In: Dusenbury C, ed. Sourcebook of bibliographic instruction. Chicago: Association of College and Research Libraries, 1993: 17-28.

8. Carson CH, Curtis RV. Applying instructional design theory to bibliographic instruction: micro theory. Res Strategies 1991 Spring;9(2)60-76.

9. Curtis RV, Carson CH. The application of motivational design to bibliographic instruction. Res Strategies 1991 Summer;9(3):130-8.

10. Carson CH, Curtis RV. Applying instructional design theory to bibliographic instruction: macro theory. Res Strategies 1991 Fall;9(4)164-79.

11. Hannum WH, Hansen C. Instructional systems development in large organizations. Englewood Cliffs, NJ: Educational Technology, 1989.

12. Lawler EE. The design of effective reward systems. In: Lorsch JW, ed. Handbook of organizational behavior. Englewood Cliffs, NJ: Prentice-Hall, 1987:225-71.

13. Shafritz JM, Koeppe RP, Soper EW. The Facts On File dictionary of education. New York: Facts On File, 1988:182-3.

14. Mager RF. Goal analysis. Belmont, CA: Fearon, 1972.

15. Fishman DL. The Maryland model statement of objectives for bibliographic instruction. Med Rèf Serv Q 1993 Summer;12(2):91-7.

16. Dusenbury C, Fusich M, Kenny K, Woodard B, eds. Read this first: an owner's guide to the new model statement of objectives for academic bibliographic instruction. Chicago: Association of College and Research Libraries, 1991.

17. Bloom BS et al., eds. Taxonomy of educational objectives: the classification of educational goals. Handbook 1: Cognitive domain. New York: David McKay, 1956.

18. Krathwohl DR, Bloom BS, Masia BB. Taxonomy of educational objectives: the classification of educational goals. Handbook 2: Affective domain. New York: David McKay, 1964.

19. Harrow AJ. A taxonomy of the psychomotor domain: a guide for developing behavioral objectives. New York: David McKay, 1972.

20. Conscious competency: the mark of a competent instructor. Personnel J 1974 Jul;53(7):538.

21. Milhollan F, Forisha BE. From Skinner to Rogers: contrasting approaches to education. Lincoln, NE: Professional Educators, 1972.

22. Ginsburg H, Opper S. Piaget's theory of intellectual development. 2d ed. Englewood Cliffs, NJ: Prentice Hall, 1979.

23. Gagne FM. The conditions of learning and theory of instruction. 4th ed. New York: Holt, Rinehart and Winston, 1985.

24. Kolb DA. Learning style inventory: self scoring inventory and interpretation booklet. Boston: McBer, 1985.

25. Bonham LA. Learning style instruments: let the buyer beware. Lifelong Learn 1988 Apr;11(6):12-6.

26. Morstain BR, Smart JC. A motivational typology of adult learners. J High Educ 1977 Nov/Dec;48(6):665-79.

27. Hensley R. Learning style theory and learning transfer principles during reference interview instruction. Libr Trends 1991 Winter;39(3):203-9.

28. Rowntree D. A dictionary of education. London: Harper & Row, 1981:86.

29. Christensen CR, Garvin DA, Sweet A, eds. Education for judgment: the artistry of discussion leadership. Boston: Harvard Business School, 1991.

30. Borgman CL. Incorporating users' information seeking styles into the design of an information retrieval interface. In: Parkhurst CA, ed. ASIS 85: proceedings of the 48th ASIS annual meeting, 1985, Las Vegas, NV, October 20-24, 1985. White Plains, NY: Knowledge Industry, 1985:324-30.

31. Stuart J, Rutherford RJD. Medical student concentration during lectures. Lancet 1978 Sep 2;2(8088):514-6.

32. Gibbs JJ. Dancing with your books: the Zen way of studying. New York: Plume, 1990.

3

Educational Programs and Materials

Melanie L. Wilson and Mary Joan (M. J.) Tooey

Librarians involved in user education are called upon to perform multifaceted tasks. They must be flexible in allocating their limited staff and time and thoughtful in designing programs that are located and scheduled conveniently. They must be both creative in selecting teaching tools and practical in designing program content with effectiveness as the primary goal. The results are user education programs that vary widely according to the particular setting, clientele, and library staff.

Conducting a target audience analysis and needs assessment, together with establishing goals and objectives, are desirable steps prior to selecting the types of programs or tools to use for library educational services. (For information on these steps, see Chapter 2 and the marketing section of Chapter 4.)

This chapter describes the broad range of educational programs available in health sciences libraries, from tours and orientations to user groups and journal clubs. Print and nonprint teaching tools are discussed in the second part of this chapter. Also noted are important considerations for successful program planning and use of materials.

Educational Programs

Tours and Orientations

Summer begins one of the busiest times of the year in many health sciences libraries. In academic and clinical settings, a new group of interns and residents arrives and, with them, a new round of library tours and orientations must be planned and conducted. As soon as these are finished, groups of new students arrive for the start of the academic year. These students bring with them the need to find information required for success in the classroom, laboratory, and clinic.

During such busy seasons, allowing tours and orientation sessions to come and go with a minimum of forethought is tempting. The world of information retrieval and management grows larger and more complex daily. Library users' demands for assistance in choosing among the many options grow as well. In contrast, one assumes that tours and orientations deal with only the most basic aspects of information management and concern the use of one specific library [1]. Tours provide answers to such questions as "Where are the photocopy machines?", "Where can I find the current issue of JAMA?", "How do I get a borrower's permit?". These questions are so commonplace that their answers may seem obvious to someone who works in the library every day. Yet a tour or orientation is frequently the user's only formal contact with a library program. The importance of this fact should not be underestimated. Faculty, administrators, and others responsible for personnel training have not always been willing to make a place for information management education in the curriculum or in the employee orientation. Even faculty and health care administrators who are astute library users may argue that curricula and workdays are already bursting. Others simply may not see the fundamental value of the skills needed to identify, locate, and use information.

When user education is assigned a standard place in the curriculum or employee training program, the time allotted may be very limited. Commonly, it is one session of short duration. What typically takes place in this time slot is the tour or orientation. This session becomes the librarian's only prescribed opportunity to convey the most essential pieces of information about the library's services and resources. In fact, the success of such a brief session may be a key factor in promoting more sophisticated subject or resource specific programs to users. Ensuring that the library tour or orientation be a valuable experience for the audience should therefore be of primary importance to librarian educators.

Goals

In practice, tours and orientations are often combined in one session. This practice has led some librarians, and users, to think of them as synonymous. Planning them separately is more effective because there is a distinct difference in their goals and the arrangements needed to make each successful.

Despite the exciting opportunities presented by the concept of the virtual library [2-3], most people associate the word *library* with a particular physical setting. Tours acquaint users with this place and with the location of materials and services in it. This goal remains largely the same for any group visiting any library. While the library may offer many kinds of programs tailored to the needs of different groups, the content of each library tour is likely to be about the same.

Unlike tours, the goals of a library orientation may change, depending on the audience. Since brevity is implied in the word *orientation,* the time typically allotted is clearly not enough to conduct in-depth instruction aimed at skill development. Still, the orientation provides an opportunity to demonstrate or describe library services or resources of particular interest to the group. This means that the content of orientations will vary.

Format

The physical arrangements for tours and orientations differ also. Tours traditionally involve groups of people following a guide through the library. The guide explains the availability and location of resources and services. Orientations, however, may take place at a location where the participants need to be seated in order to observe a demonstration, see an overhead projection, or examine a print resource.

A large tour group is likely to create a disturbance for other users as the participants congregate. Meeting the group outside the library entrance or in a meeting room within the library is desirable. If a lockable meeting room is available, consider beginning the session there, so that participants do not have to carry their belongings with them. It is uncomfortable, distracting, and difficult for the visitor to listen effectively while constantly moving a heavy backpack from shoulder to shoulder or juggling a coat and briefcase.

Handouts associated with tours, such as maps and library guidebooks, are best distributed at the beginning of the tour. The guide can then make reference to them without disrupting the flow of the presentation to hand them out. In contrast, handouts for orientations may prove distracting to participants if all are distributed at the beginning of the session. A better choice is to hand them out at appropriate times during the presentation.

While conducting a group from site to site in the library, the guide should wait at each stop until all participants have arrived before speaking to the group. The guide should inform participants at the beginning of each session as to how questions will be handled. If time allows, the guide can invite participants to satisfy their curiosity by asking questions at any time during the session. If the schedule is tight, one can ask the group for questions at a few specified points on the tour.

Noise is an incendiary issue in some libraries. Posting the library tour schedule well in advance will alert users that the library may be noisy during those times. Notifying users ten minutes before the tour begins, by a walk-through announcement or use of the public address system, can be a politic thing to do. Explaining to tour participants that the noise carries in the library will encourage their cooperation during the tour, and their understanding as future users.

Content

Knowledge of the characteristics of the audience and its expectations is vital to the planning of meaningful user education programs. Organizing the content of the tour or orientation can begin after this information is collected and understood. (For more information on characteristics of adult learners and target audience analysis, see Chapter 2. For a description of needs assessment, see Chapter 4.)

The content should be limited to those components most relevant to the group, presented in the most appropriate manner. The introduction to a tour or orientation, and any other user education program, includes several elements:

- Introduction of the library staff member.
- Introduction of the participants.
- Objectives of the session.
- Logistics of the session.

Logistics include any of the format items described in the previous section, as well as a brief description of how the time will be spent.

The following points might be covered in a library tour:

- Parking, transportation, or other accessibility considerations related to the library.
- Entrances and exits to the library. This may seem obvious, but is not always. At the Hardin Library for the Health Sciences at the University of Iowa, for example, one enters and exits the library building on the third floor.
- Number of floors, rooms, or basic arrangement of the library.
- Important signs or landmarks within the library.

- Location of essential library services and how to obtain them, e.g, circulation, reference, photocopying, database searching, interlibrary loan.
- Essential library resources and use requirements: journal collection, books, audiovisuals, library catalog, microcomputers, reserve materials, reference collection.
- Where to obtain additional information, for example, information desks, print and nonprint guides, telephone numbers.

An orientation might include the following:

- Description of the services most relevant to the needs of a particular group, e.g., reference consultations, user education programs, table of contents services, Literature Attached to the CHart (LATCH) programs, database searching services.
- Instruction in the use of the library's catalog, journal holdings lists, or other locator tools.
- A look at specific collections of interest, e.g., the rare book room for history of medicine students.
- Some elements of bibliographic instruction to pique the participants' interest to learn more, for example, how to read a citation or a brief introduction to a pertinent index.

For more ideas on designing effective orientations, see the references listed at the end of this chapter [4-6].

Liaison and Clinical Medical Librarian Programs

A liaison program is established when a librarian is assigned to a particular school, program, or service to

- Develop knowledge about the curriculum or major aspects of the program or service.
- Meet the instructional needs of that group of users.

The librarian may also have collection development responsibilities and act as a conduit for the exchange of information between the library and the school, program, or service. Liaisons are often invited to serve on committees with these users. Through this personal interaction, liaisons gain knowledge about specific library education needs. The librarian is then able to approach faculty or administrators in a proactive manner to offer education and training.

In the hospital setting, the clinical medical librarian (CML) is the equivalent of the liaison. A personal relationship is also an important part of a CML program. The concept originally evolved in the hospital library setting. It was seen as a way for the librarian to be an integral part of the health care team by providing information when and where it was needed [7]. By attending medical and surgical rounds and responding to clinical questions with informational support, the librarian is able to take the library to the health care professional. As CML programs have evolved, new educational roles have been undertaken. These include providing database training and searching support [8-9]. The roles of collection developer and research partner have also been assumed [10-11].

Point-of-Need Assistance

Point-of-need assistance is available from two sources: library staff and supporting materials. Library staff provide point-of-need assistance to a user when they respond to a specific request at the time and place that help is required. The information professional then has a wonderful opportunity to provide instruction based on the user's need to know [12]. Providing such personal assistance is usually the responsibility of reference staff.

Because staff assistance is labor intensive and often in high demand, libraries may need to establish service policies. How much time can be spent on requests, or what level of assistance can be given to an individual user during busy periods, are examples of this type of guideline.

In addition to one-on-one instruction, many libraries provide point-of-need assistance via print and nonprint materials. These are discussed later in this chapter under educational materials.

Consultation

A consultation service takes point-of-need instruction one step further. A librarian meets with an individual or small group regarding a specific information request. The librarian may provide coaching on a broad range of topics:

- Organizing a search for information.
- Selecting appropriate print and nonprint resources.
- Describing or demonstrating how to use the resources.
- Managing or organizing the information found [13-14].

For example, a nursing student working on a master's thesis might request a consultation to get personalized advice on conducting a literature search on the thesis topic. A clinician may ask for advice in choosing software to control a reprint collection.

With careful planning and advertising, a consultation service need not overwhelm the library staff. Two general guidelines are suggested.

- First, making consultations available by appointment is advisable. This procedure allows the consultation to be scheduled with the staff member who has the most expertise in the specified subject area. Advance scheduling also ensures that the user will have the librarian's undivided attention.
- Second, the user should be asked for a brief description of the request topic when the appointment is made. The librarian will then have the information needed to prepare materials in advance and organize a thoughtful response to the request.

Staffing for consultations can be effectively linked with a library liaison program. For example, in an academic setting, it might be most appropriate for a pharmacy student to consult with the liaison librarian for the pharmacy program. This is a benefit for the library, as well as the user, since the liaisons gain information concerning programs, curricula, and research within their areas of responsibility.

Librarians can also serve as information consultants for special projects or for officially designated groups within the institution, thus bringing more relevant and timely information to these groups. This type of consulting also provides an opportunity to educate other members of the organization about the services of the library. The abilities that library staff can bring to the research, educational, or patient care activities of the institution are highlighted.

Consulting with users can provide a wealth of data about how clinicians, nurses, researchers, and others find and use information in their day-to-day lives. These observations can be used to improve or expand all library services.

Bibliographic Instruction

The information-related activities in which health sciences librarians are commonly involved form a continuum. This continuum extends from the clarification of an information need; to the effective use of appropriate sources of information to fill the need; to the organization, management, and application of the information to the original problem.

Bibliographic instruction, often referred to as BI by librarians, focuses on the middle part of this construct—the effective use of appropriate resources. Its primary objective goes beyond making users aware of the existence of particular library resources; that may have been accomplished in an orientation session. BI's main objective is to help users develop skill in using resources effectively. A prime example of a bibliographic instruction session is a program to teach citation verification and interlibrary loan procedures to secretaries and research assistants [15].

In terms of content, BI sessions are often discipline or resource specific, e.g., "How to Use CINAHL," "Library Resources for Dentists," or "Searching *Index Medicus* for Information." The resources covered have traditionally been print or audiovisual. Today, BI sessions often include instruction on the use of CD-ROM, online, or other electronic equivalents of print tools. Although the format of the tools has changed, the focus of BI is still bibliographic information.

BI sessions differ from consultations in that they generally involve librarian interaction with a group. Hands-on use of the information tools is a desirable component for skill development, and a part of a galaxy of teaching methods used in bibliographic instruction.

Information Management Education

The goal of information management education (IME) programs is to increase the independence and confidence levels of health care professionals relative to information seeking. These programs are proactive and collaborative [16]. IME

> ...refers to instructing users in the identification, retrieval, evaluation, and use of information...[it] demands that librarians instruct users in how to use and manage information, departing from their traditional role as mere providers [17].

IME sessions can include the following:

- Training end users to search computerized resources.
- Describing and demonstrating software or systems that might be used for literature searching.
- Showing how to use bibliographic file management software.
- Teaching critical analysis of the literature.
- Teaching how to access Internet resources via gophers.

As this list suggests, IME tries to expand users' knowledge of information sources beyond the library's walls. One example is educational support of computer conferencing [18]. Teaching the use of gophers and wide area information services (WAIS) is another example [19-20]. Gophers are a type of software that provides flexible menu-format access to Internet resources. The software is named after the Gopher system developed at the University of Minnesota [21]. WAIS is client-server software that provides a common interface for searching distributed databases. Bibliographic, full-text, and factual databases can all be searched with the same interface, regardless of the databases' individual search protocols [22].

The content and format of IME sessions are varied. Buchanan and Fazzone describe some in the hospital setting [23]. Many use hands-on experience with print resources, microcomputer hardware, and software. These sessions usually take place in a classroom or microcomputer laboratory.

Class- or Course-Related Instruction

Class-related library instruction is often initiated by faculty members who need help from the library to enable their students to complete assignments or research papers specific to their courses. The instruction usually takes place during regularly scheduled class time, either in the classroom or in the library. This type of instruction meets a specific and time-sensitive need. The class is tailored to meet that need and may involve multiple resources. The potential exists for class-related instruction to become a long-term commitment. Faculty members may build library classes into their courses every time they are offered, especially if curriculum-integrated instruction is not available.

Curriculum-Integrated Instruction

Within the academic health sciences center, perhaps the area that has seen the largest growth in the last few years is that of curricular integration of information management skills. Curricular integration involves designing an entire course of study that builds an individual's information identification, acquisition, and management skills. The course of study goes on to help students synthesize these abilities to support lifelong learning.

Study of these skills becomes an integral part of the curriculum in one of three ways. The first is for the course of study to be a required program that all students must take, as they would a core course like biochemistry [24]. The second is for the information management course to be offered as an elective and open to all students in all programs [25]. The third integrates information management skills in a series of courses, with progressively more complex skills taught throughout the students' academic program [26], either through elective or required courses [27]. Some of the topics to be covered in instruction of this type might include the following:

- The structure of knowledge.
  Where information comes from.
  How it is organized and disseminated.
  In what formats it exists.
- How to obtain information.
  Manually and electronically.
  As an end user.
  Through information professionals.
- Management of the information.
  Manual file systems.
  Reprint file software.
- Integration and future access.
  Critical analysis.
  Journal article publication.

The curriculum might also focus on specific resources applicable to the local setting, for example, electronic patient care notebooks.

The biggest roadblock to any type of curricular integration is the inflexibility of many current curricula; there simply is no room for adding a program of this type. A critical opportunity exists for librarians when a curriculum is about to undergo a review or revision. Having an effective means of providing input to the reviewing body, either through membership or by representation, is extremely important [28].

One recent trend that has added impetus to the integration of information management education into health sciences curricula is problem-based learning [29-30]. Advocates of this learning model argue that students learn best when presented with a problem to solve. As the students approach their problem—which is often a clinical diagnostic or therapeutic situation—they must effectively use a variety of information sources to solve the problem. This learning model is very information dependent. The availability and use of all manner of problem-related information becomes very important to the students. For example, when presented with a laboratory value, the student may need to use library resources to determine what the value indicates. As they reach a diagnosis or ponder treatment options, they may need the support of a literature review to verify their conclusions. The library can also supply background data that may be needed if the student is asked to present the case to a group. As more health sciences institutions embrace problem-based learning, the educational role of the library can be expanded, and curricular integration becomes more of a possibility. These opportunities are described in the literature [31].

Curricular integration must be backed by library administration, academic faculty, and the administrators of the school or program. Library administrators must acknowledge the amount of staff time and effort likely to be required by a project of this type, and find means of supporting that effort. Also, without promotion by academic administrators and faculty who see it as an integral part of education, there is little chance that an information management curriculum will gain acceptance by the students.

The planning steps taken to integrate library instruction into the curriculum should involve academic administrators, faculty, students, and library staff, so that the curriculum will meet the expectations of everyone involved. After the initial meetings, it is important to set goals for the program, set objectives for each session, establish the content of the individual sessions, flesh out the session, plan for supplemental materials, develop the syllabus, and decide how the students will be evaluated. In addition to measuring student achievement, provisions must be made for evaluating the success of the curriculum itself and assessing whether or not programmatic goals have been reached. (For more information about these steps, see Chapter 5.)

Health Informatics Curricula

Some librarians are involved in teaching basic computer literacy with applications programs such as word processors and spreadsheets. Sometimes these skills are taught as part of a health informatics curriculum. These curricula include instruction in the use of advanced technologies to synthesize and manage clinical information [32]. Librarians should investigate partnerships with the faculty in these types of programs, since the acquisition and management of information is not only a primary function of libraries, but a cornerstone of the informatics curriculum. If a partnership is developed between informatics and library instruction, students will have an opportunity to learn knowledge management skills from the creation of information to its application at the patient bedside.

The prospect of having a long-term impact on the attitudes and behavior of health sciences students is an exciting point for instructional librarians to consider. Only carefully framed studies will tell whether or not this type of instruction has an effect on the quality of patient care.

User Groups and Journal Clubs

User groups are collections of individuals sharing common interests in a technology or skill. The groups conduct business entirely electronically or combine electronic communication with meetings and other organized activities [33-34]. Health sciences libraries have sponsored groups specializing in end-user searching, database management, educational applications of computers, and others [35]. The activities these groups undertake include

- Maintaining electronic bulletin boards or computer conferences.
- Sponsoring workshops and product demonstrations.
- Exchanging user aids, public domain software, and shareware.
- Answering questions and sharing ideas.
- Assembling membership directories.
- Compiling articles or bibliographies on topics of general interest to members.
- Conducting software or hardware evaluations.
- Promoting consumer advocacy.
- Publishing newsletters.

The primary benefits to participants are camaraderie and information and resource sharing.

Journal clubs provide similar opportunities for discussion and learning. They tend to be focused on keeping apprised of the literature in the group's area of interest, but some cover other information formats such as video [36]. The purposes of journal clubs include one or more of the following:

- Serve as a current awareness forum.
- Increase knowledge on a particular topic.
- Develop skill in critical analysis of the literature [37-38].

The factors associated with successful journal clubs and user groups appear to be the same: regularly scheduled meetings, congenial atmosphere, shared responsibility for programs, mutual respect among members, and a focus on real needs [39-40].

The creativity of librarians in addressing the specific educational needs of their users has produced many permutations on the types of programs described here. User groups and journal clubs are just examples of adapting user education to new environments.

Educational Materials

As discussed in Chapter 2, most adults have personal learning styles which have been developed over time. Some users may learn and retain information better through reading print materials, some through observation, some aurally, some through hands-on interaction, and some through a combination of sensory paths. Selecting which materials and techniques to use in a particular program will depend on many factors. Devising appropriate teaching materials is a challenge that calls upon the ingenuity and resourcefulness of those designing user education experiences. (For a list of sources of materials, see Appendix B.)

A particular challenge for librarians involved in user education is how to effectively respond to a request to provide instruction for a large group. It may be impossible to provide tours for the entire first-year class of medical students, for example, especially if the time frame involved is one hour on one specific day. Ironically, the formats that provide a partial solution to this problem are also a reasonable response to a situation on the opposite end of the spectrum—providing convenient instruction for individual users who request it. There are several advantages to making a variety of self-directed instructional materials available to users:

- Interesting self-directed materials can be alternatives or adjuncts to formal instruction.
- The user can go over the information as often as desired.
- The program assures that every person using it receives the same information presented in the same way.
- Scheduling and allocating time for an instructional session become the responsibility of the interested user or group.
- The guidance of library staff is not required.
- Some formats do not require the user or group to come to the library, which may be an advantage when the group is located at a distance from the building.

The above advantages must be weighed against users not having direct, personal contact with a library staff member. Some users feel this is depersonalizing [41].

The following section describes materials that are appropriate for use both in formal educational settings and for self-directed learning. These range from signs and a printed walking tour of the library to a sophisticated hypertext tutorial explaining how to use a particular resource.

Exhibits

Library exhibits can be very effective educational tools. Their ability to accommodate realia gives them potentially greater impact and flexibility than signs, posters, and other two-dimensional library materials. Typically, exhibits do not showcase long textual passages; rather, the viewer learns primarily through graphics and displayed objects.

Focusing on a single theme and arranging the material so the display appears orderly and uncluttered are important. Exhibits or displays can be shown on bulletin boards, in glassed-in cabinets, or on tables. It is helpful to plan the exhibit to scale on graph paper to ensure that everything will fit within the area allotted [42-43].

If there is no time or budget to produce in-house displays, the National Library of Medicine or one of the Regional Medical Libraries may be of help in identifying traveling exhibits that are available for loan. Other sources for exhibits include faculty members who might want to showcase private collections. Departments or schools that are celebrating anniversaries or special accomplishments are another source. The library is often a perfect central location for disseminating information through exhibits.

Print Materials

When microcomputers appeared on the scene and proliferated in educational institutions, print materials fell somewhat out of favor. Computer-based instruction was not always warranted, but the allure of technology was very hard for many instructional designers to resist.

Desktop publishing, with its ease of use and wide availability, has made print an acceptable instructional form again. A firm grasp of visual design skills, including appropriate use of text, graphics, and page layout, is needed to be successful at designing print materials.

Print materials are very effective for adults who want highly transportable education or who are not comfortable with computer technology. Curling up by a fire with a laptop computer does not have the same affective results for most people as doing so with print media. The purpose of this section is to describe important aspects in the production of print materials, and the most common forms they may take.

Authorship

While design, layout, and production of library materials should be supervised or coordinated by one person or department, authorship is logically dependent on the content and scope of the material. Each guide should be critiqued by one or more reviewers before it goes to press. The reviewers should be less familiar with the topic than the author, so they can identify any problems a library novice might encounter in its use. The reviewers should also look for problems of organization, writing style, design, and production. In addition, all print materials should be examined on a regular basis, at least twice a year, to reevaluate usefulness and to spot needed revisions. Such analysis is an essential element in the production of print materials.

Design and Production

Print materials should be kept simple and uncluttered. Since a library's publications represent it in the eyes of its users, design and production should receive careful attention. These should contribute not only to the utility of the document, but to a positive impression consistent with the image of the library. Some may argue over just how far such efforts should go, i.e., how slick such publications need appear. For example, library guides are developed primarily for utility. Library users look for them and use them, but generally do not place a high value on them. It can be argued that their production quality need not be as high as that required for the library's annual report.

Certain minimum standards should be defined library-wide, however. Consistency in paper color, type font, logo, and other design elements will unite the materials visually. Uniform design elements will aid users in identifying library publications in general and various kinds of guides in particular.

The following are suggested minimum standards:

- Well-written, logically organized content, free of library jargon.
- Attractive layout that assists use of the guide.
- Clear printing in an easy-to-read typeface.
- Paper which holds ink well.
- Paper color that provides an easy-to-read contrast to the printing.

Design and production of print materials may be improved greatly through the use of desktop publishing and file management software. These are useful for laying out graphics and text attractively for both print and computer-based tools. Word processing has made both producing and updating them an easy task. Even if print materials are sent outside the library to be reproduced, the text can be maintained in-house and easily changed.

It is usually better and cheaper to print smaller quantities of brochures so that large quantities of incorrect or out-of-date brochures do not accumulate. This method is especially true for volatile topics such as remote access to campus or institutional information resources. Although printing smaller numbers may appear to be more costly, on a per-unit basis, it will not be the case if the library must throw away a large quantity of outdated material.

Printing in volume must also be weighed against the time spent in correcting brochures or inadvertently distributing erroneous information. Inserts for brochures can be used for information that changes. For example, an insert could be used to list a schedule of classes that varies over the course of the year.

Creating print materials can be labor intensive and expensive. The flexibility of utilities such as HyperCard, however, can provide both a means of production for the librarian and an efficient interactive program for the user. Hypertext and hypermedia software are described later in this chapter.

Types of Print Materials

Signs

The value of signs as an educational tool cannot be overstated. Effective signs may be the only type of instruction some library users need. The major objectives of signs, whether or not they are part of a library-wide graphics plan, are

1. They point users to locations where additional help is available from library staff.
2. They direct users to resources, such as the current journals or the reference collection.
3. They inform users about library policies and procedures in a very direct and public way.
4. Signs of a temporary nature, such as posters, can be used to advertise library programs.

Like other kinds of print materials, signs are especially valuable because they quickly answer a user's question and reduce the need for staff to handle simple, recurring queries.

In general, permanent signs should be planned and produced as a group, to ensure consistency in wording and appearance. Time and cost-benefit factors are likely to be the major determinants of the quality of permanent signs.

Entire volumes have been written on library signs and several sources are listed at the end of this chapter. Johnson's article is a particularly good summary and contains a helpful bibliography [44-47]. Three important elements of effective signs are discussed here.

Message

The message, most often expressed in words, should be concise, clear, and free of jargon. Spell out abbreviations which may be obscure, e.g., Interlibrary Loan rather than ILL. Signs that convey their message by use of symbols may also be effective, providing the symbols are universally understood by the user group.

Legibility and Readability

Most importantly, the sign should be easy to read. Several factors contribute to legibility and readability. The length of the message should fit the size of the sign so that it appears uncluttered. A simple type font, such as Roman, is better than an elaborate one. The size of the lettering should be suitable for the distance from which the sign will be viewed. Background and lettering colors should be combined to please the eye and provide enough contrast for easy reading.

Location

Signs should be placed in such a way that the view of their surface is unobstructed. Lighting should be adequate for reading without glare. This is especially important if the sign is intended to be viewed from a distance.

Signs act as an institutional signature; their appearance reflects on the library, as does the appearance of other printed library materials. Care should be taken, therefore, to plan and maintain signs that are effective, clean, and professional in appearance. Those made from wood or plastic are often the most aesthetically pleasing and long-wearing.

Although hand lettering may be needed for temporary signs, it is usually harder to read and may reflect poorly on the library. A preferable alternative to hand lettering is the use of computer software specifically designed for making signs. These programs are available in various price ranges and levels of sophistication, including shareware programs such as SIGN. The size of the paper that the printer can handle defines the size of the signs. Used with a laser printer, these programs can often produce signs with good print quality.

Brief Guide

Library guides are a common, relatively inexpensive educational service for any library to provide. Such guides have traditionally been available in print format. The capabilities and widespread availability of computers has led many libraries to also make such guides available electronically.

The brief guide aims to describe succinctly the library's services and resources. This document may list

- The library's location.
- Library hours.
- Various departments and phone numbers.
- Brief explanations of library policies, such as borrower registration.
- Size and scope of the collection.

The brief guide may also include a map of the library. Such guides are extremely useful adjuncts to library orientations and tours, providing a summary of the session for future reference.

A brief guide should be no longer than both sides of one sheet of paper. There are two reasons for this. Since the whole intent of this guide is to provide a brief, general overview, the document should be short. Secondly, since the guide will be valuable for almost all library users, it will be necessary to print and distribute more copies of this document than perhaps any other item. For the sake of economy, the simpler and cheaper the guide is to reproduce, the better.

Printed Tour

A printed walking tour of the library is sometimes combined with a brief guide. Users follow a printed map that leads them along a certain route through the library. It provides information on various important stops along the way. Such tours cost little to produce and are easily updated. However, they require the user to constantly look up and down from the printed sheet. This may be acceptable for individuals, but is cumbersome for groups.

Library Newsletter

The library newsletter can be an effective part of user education. It provides a regular forum for communicating important information about library resources and services. If the library can mail the newsletter or distribute it electronically, users who cannot visit the library in person can be kept up-to-date [48].

Most library newsletters are from two to eight pages in length. There are many sources of help in putting a newsletter together. Chris Olson & Associates produces a quarterly publication, *Assistant Editor,* which contains articles and library artwork that can be adapted or placed directly in one's own newsletter. Subscribers own the copyright to the material, which is available in print or electronic form. There is help in the literature, as well [49-51].

Library Handbook

A library handbook is an in-depth document for users planning to do extensive library research. It is also valuable for library trustees, institutional administrators, or others whose interest requires more detail. As well as providing complete information on services, it may describe the library's administrative structure, its collections, staff, and technological resources.

Programmed Texts and Workbooks

Print materials include programmed instructional texts and workbooks, both of which can be self-paced. Programmed texts tend to provide immediate feedback through the use of self-testing, while workbooks tend to be less rigorous instructionally. Programmed texts test users on small, distinct portions of information before the user goes on to the next segment. "It is especially appropriate for highly detailed and closely sequenced content that can be broken down into individual units of information" [52]. There are commercially available programmed texts and workbooks that can be used as is or adapted to the local setting.

Specialized Guides

There are three types of specialized guides: point-of-use, pathfinders, and policy-related documents.

Point-of-Use Guides

Point-of-use guides provide instruction at a particular site within the library. An example is a card affixed to a public terminal, describing how to search the online catalog for a title. Point-of-use materials are usually in print form. They are designed to instruct users concerning a particular tool such as an index or CD-ROM workstation. Point-of-use materials should accurately represent what users will see when using the resource and illustrate solutions to common problems. Keeping the guides up-to-date is important. In writing and designing point-of-use materials, the following guidelines should be kept in mind:

- Answer the most common questions, but keep it simple. The user should not be overwhelmed by detail.
- If using the resource is a multistep process, break the process down into logical segments.
- List other resources or persons who can provide additional help or more information.

Point-of-use guides can also be created in a nonprint format using any number of the tools described later in this chapter [53].

Pathfinders

A second type of guide is sometimes called a pathfinder. This guide suggests ways to identify and locate materials in a specific subject area or type of publication. Examples are guides on how to find information on environmental health or how to find patents. The format and guidelines for developing these have been described in the literature [54-56].

Policy-Related Documents

The third type of guide clearly explains the library's policies. An example is a bookmarker or library card stating the loan periods for journals.

All of these specialized guides contribute to the library's educational program in several important ways:

- They can answer highly specific questions without the involvement of a staff member.
- They can serve as useful adjuncts to library instruction by summarizing the content of a session.
- They provide a public, written statement of library policies, a useful clarification for both users and staff.
- They provide inexpensive materials which library users can take with them for later reference.

Distribution

For the above reasons, it behooves librarians to display print materials prominently and be generous in their distribution. Having a central location for all the library's publications is especially important. It helps users find specific guides, see others that may be of interest, and aids staff in answering questions. Additional copies of specific guides can also be made available at the appropriate service and resource sites in the library. Customized packets can be assembled for various groups and distributed by mail or at the beginning of user education programs. At the University of Maryland, the full text of all library brochures is available on UMABnet, the campus gopher system. The availability of new library guides should be announced in the library's newsletter, at a minimum.

Nonprint Tools

Nonprint teaching tools can include sound, visual effects, and hands-on interactions that provide users with a richer educational experience. Such enrichment is especially important when the materials are being used by individuals or groups when a library staff member is not present.

Nonprint teaching materials do not need to be produced in-house. Many options exist for borrowing, renting, and purchasing materials. *The Video Source Book*, published annually by Gale Research, indexes videotapes by subject and includes producer name and purchase price [57]. With information from *The Video Source Book*, a librarian can opt to contact the producer directly to arrange for purchase or rental, when available. Searching for these videos on OCLC will show if they are available through interlibrary loan for use or preview.

Many professional associations, such as the American Management Association or the American Physical Therapy Association, make available nonprint materials that are relevant to some user education programs. AVLINE, produced by the National Library of Medicine (NLM), is a bibliographic database of audiovisual materials. It is accessible through the MEDLARS system by modem or through the NLM Locator system on the Internet. (For other sources of nonprint tools, see Appendix B.)

Nonprint materials are not always readily available. The following sections discuss some points to consider when producing them.

Authorship

The production of nonprint materials may require the expertise of persons not directly involved in user education. Production is often a cooperative project between those with technological expertise and those with content expertise. Content experts decide the educational objectives to be met. As with print resources, each production should be critiqued by one or more outside reviewers during the production process, to identify any problems a user might encounter with it. The reviewers should look for problems related to sound and visual clarity, organization of content, and overall effectiveness.

Production

Before producing an audiovisual or computer-assisted teaching tool, the user education librarian should have a clear idea of the educational objectives to be met by the finished product. No level of sophistication will make up for a production that is without focus. After establishing objectives, one can decide what format will most effectively suit the objectives and content. If one would like to have a tour of the library available when a librarian is absent, an audiotaped walking tour will be sufficient. However, if the objective is to provide a physical orientation to the library for those outside the library setting, then a videotape will be much more appropriate.

Once the format is chosen, the content can be organized. In cases where there is a visual component, the librarian should sketch the sequence of visual events. This sketch is a drawn plan, or storyboard, showing what will appear with the audio component. The storyboard should include notes about any desired lighting, visual composition, or other photographic considerations. (For more information on instructional design, see Chapter 2.)

Types of Nonprint Materials

Audiotape

Audiotaped instruction is most effective when accompanied by slides, a printed script, or some other visual aid. This format has the potential for being more enjoyable and informative for the user than a print counterpart. However, it is much more complicated to produce and update. Audiotaped instruction is most suitable for individual use.

Transparencies

Transparencies can be functional tools in formal user education programs. They are not suitable for self-directed programs since they are not, by themselves, either engaging or informative enough to be effective. Production of such materials has been greatly simplified by sheets of transparency film that can be run through a photocopy machine. All that is needed for production is a printed master and a supply of blank transparencies.

For readability, the image shown must contrast strongly with the background color of the transparency. This contrast is especially important in settings where the ambient lighting is not fully adjustable. Also, it is preferable to break the content down and use several transparencies to convey a message. This procedure allows the designer to use larger print on each, making the transparencies easier to read and more attractive.

Slides

The versatility of slides makes them a very useful teaching tool. Simply rearranging the slides or selecting certain ones can result in several effective packages for different teaching situations.

An important first step in production is making a storyboard showing what information or image each slide will contain. Some slides may need to be professionally produced. However, most can be made using a computer to produce the images and an attached camera to photograph them. This has simplified the slide-making process.

A less expensive, "low tech" way to produce some slides is to have interested library staff take the photographs, using a standard 35-mm camera with slide film. Acceptable results for interior shots, other than close-ups, can often be achieved in this manner. Following a few basic principles will ensure the best results: keep the shot simple, use appropriate lighting, and center the subject.

Slide/Tape

Slide/tape programs are useful for orientations that introduce the user to the library's services and resources. They are less effective than other formats in orienting users to the library building because it is difficult to convey directions. If converted to videotape, and edited for this purpose, this drawback can be overcome.

Attractive and moderate in cost to produce, slide/tape is one of the few answers to orienting a large group located at a distance from the library. These programs are also useful for groups with a very limited amount of time to spend on library-related instruction.

Without a library staff member in attendance, synchronizing the display of the slides with the taped narration can be a problem. One solution is to videotape a slide/tape presentation. The videotape is also easier to update.

Videotape

The ability of video to present moving pictures and a less stilted overall presentation makes it more visually attractive than slide/tape programs. Videotape has become a common delivery system for all types of instruction, even though its use is sometimes inappropriate. Usually, video is found to be productive when affective objectives are to be met, for example, to motivate the target audience. Video is also effective when a consistent message needs to be delivered to a large group over a period of time.

Video is not recommended as the primary technique for teaching psychomotor skills because practice, repetition, and feedback are required to master these skills. However, video can be useful as part of a larger learning system for skills training.

Videotapes can also be useful for orienting users located at a distance from the library building. Unfortunately, this format is also more costly and complicated to produce than a slide/tape program.

Creating an effective videotape instructional module requires special skills, including scriptwriting, visual design skills, an understanding of how to interpret a concept using video, and editing skills. All of the production elements mentioned earlier in this chapter should be considered. Other design elements to be weighed include sound and visual clarity, speed of presentation, and length of the finished product.

Care must be taken to assure that the information to be communicated comes across on the screen. Many people assume that developing an instructional video is no more complicated than shooting a home video. Educational services librarians contemplating the production of instructional videos need to be aware of the differences between professional and amateur techniques [58].

On many campuses and in many hospitals, there are audiovisual or art departments that can assist the librarian in producing instructional videotapes. If these types of services are not available, private videographers can help. In any case, *Creative Approaches to Video for Bibliographic Instruction* will be of use to library staff who contemplate being producers or scriptwriters [59]. Some of the reasons for choosing a videotape format, planning concerns, and a cost analysis are presented by Shedlock and Tawyea [60].

Computer-Based Formats

Advances in microcomputer, laser disc, and electronic file transfer technology have increased the options for self-directed instruction. These advancements have many interesting applications in user education. Having instruction available on diskette makes library programs easily portable for use on compatible equipment outside the library. Similarly, individual screens can be printed and used as handouts or made into transparencies. The sophisticated graphics created with such programs can make for a very engaging instructional package. However, these programs can be labor intensive to produce from scratch and therefore more costly than some of the print options.

Libraries with online catalogs or local area networks can now distribute library information in electronic form through these systems. Users of the University of Iowa's OASIS online catalog and information system, for example, can type "exp hours" at any command screen to see the hours for the various university libraries. This distribution method is convenient to both in-house users and those who may access the library catalog via modem or other means.

Computer-Assisted Instruction (CAI)

Also known as computer-based training (CBT), CAI enables independent learning about a specific topic by incorporating instruction, evaluation, and feedback in a computer program. Computer-assisted instruction is an effective, interactive, transportable delivery system for people comfortable with computers. It is useful for those who enjoy learning at their own pace and for those who do not require or want the social interactions provided by group instruction. Other factors that favor CAI applications are described by Turner [61].

CAI can be created by using authoring systems. These systems are specialized computer software that allow instructional designers to create interactive teaching programs using established protocols. Advanced programming skills are not required. Authoring systems are available for both MS-DOS and Macintosh. In some cases, programs developed in one environment can be converted to the other environment.

While a novice can learn to use an authoring system, a sophisticated understanding of visual and verbal communication is required to produce a program that effectively meets stated instructional objectives. Unfortunately, many CAI programs are primarily text—automated page turners with little value added beyond that of a printed textbook. These fail to use the capabilities of CAI. Good CAI is based on good instructional design, just as with any effective teaching. There are excellent guides available that explain how to harness the power of the computer for instruction [62]. Local colleges and universities often have experts available for consultation, as well.

Because the price of designing a constructive computer-assisted instruction program is high, only topics that are somewhat static are good candidates for this medium. The cost of frequent revisions is prohibitive. As with video, using CAI to teach psychomotor skills is not recommended unless the CAI is a piece of a monitored multipart instructional system.

Some libraries are now using computer-assisted instruction to replace other passive and more labor and materials intensive modes of instruction. The Bio-Agricultural Library at the University of California, Riverside, uses CAI to introduce students to the online catalog and two major literature indexes. The library formerly used lectures, tours, workbooks, and in-library exercises to teach this material [63]. Although not many of these applications have been in health sciences libraries, they are useful examples of CAI's capabilities.

Hypertext

Hypertext programs are computerized text-retrieval interfaces that allow easy maneuverability between sets of screens through the use of an on-screen pointer. For example, a library user can look at the library floor plan on one screen. By moving the mouse attachment on the computer, the user can move the cursor to the information desk shown on the floor plan. By clicking the mouse on the information desk symbol, the user can then see a screen describing the services and materials provided there.

Hypertext software also allows for the easy addition, deletion, or reconfiguration of such screens. HyperCard, an Apple program developed for the Macintosh, is an example of this type of software. The University of Maryland at Baltimore created the Electronic Guide And Directory (EGAD) with HyperCard. The program uses the graphics capabilities of the software for maps and answers basic directional questions. The Computer-Aided Reference station (CAR) program developed at the University of Tennessee at Memphis is another attempt to provide a workstation to aid in the use of the library [64].

Hypertext programs can be attached to peripheral devices such as CD-ROM, videodisc, videotape players, or slide/tape equipment. This combination of visual, voice, and text materials related to a particular subject is known as hypermedia or multimedia.

Multimedia

Simply stated, multimedia is the integration of computer, text, graphics, animation, and sound [65]. Multimedia programs can be developed in any computer environment, but the most effective software currently exists for Macintosh and MS-DOS [66]. There is a legitimate argument to be made that multimedia is nothing more than a new name for computer-assisted instruction. Well-designed CAI would take advantage of all the capabilities of the computer that were appropriate for the specific instructional task. This would make a good CAI program indistinguishable from what is currently being labeled multimedia.

Videodisc

Inexpensive videodisc playback equipment has created new opportunities for librarian educators. Videodisc technology is a superior storage medium for a large number of still images, can incorporate rolling video and sound, and can also incorporate computer programs to drive and control the instructional system. Videodiscs can be used by individuals or small groups of students learning at their own pace, or they can be used by an instructor to illustrate lectures.

Videodisc is a potent independent learning tool. A single learner using a customized bar-coded workbook can be prompted through a learning sequence and even receive feedback. While videodisc development is enormously expensive, creating workbooks to be used with existing videodiscs is very cost-effective. Because there are large numbers of videodiscs on the market that have a medical content, use of this tool is both feasible and advisable for educational services librarians [67]. An example of discs available in the medical library realm are the Slice of Life discs developed by the University of Utah [68].

One disadvantage of this technology, besides development cost, is the expense of distributing the discs and equipment at sites convenient to learners. In most cases, the learner's work site is best. Librarians can provide workstations in the library or at selected remote locations to help learners become comfortable with the technology and encourage its adoption. People's reluctance to use this new technology can be overcome with techniques for diffusing innovation [69].

Expert Systems

Expert systems and neural networks are another interesting computer-based tool that can be adapted for instruction. Because these programs are complex, both in design and execution, they are computer driven. Expert systems are essentially decision trees. They attempt to mimic standard decision-making processes through the use of elaborate sets of rules [70]. Neural networks expand on this concept and reduce the need for massive rule structures by providing sets of heuristics that the program uses to make judgments in the decision process. Simple expert systems developed by librarians have provided assistance with basic information needs, such as helping users identify an appropriate index for a literature search [71-72].

Expert systems and neural networks are expensive to produce but hold great promise for circumventing some of the complexity of information retrieval systems. When a library user needs to find specific information and is faced with dozens of indexes, a well-designed expert system can help the user make a reasonable choice [73]. At the National Library of Medicine (NLM), a MEDSTATS program is being developed to enable the user to find references to English-language monographs and monographic series volumes in the NLM collection that contain specific statistics. The user can then telephone or e-mail NLM to have a reference librarian look up the statistic. MEDSTATS does not provide the actual statistics.

There are additional models of programs in nursing, medicine, and other health disciplines that go beyond drill and practice instruction. These programs present clinical simulations, which offer opportunities for the user to react to real clinical problems, make diagnostic decisions, and experience the consequences of those decisions. These programs often integrate the computer with audio and video recorded on a laser disc. These models can be used by librarians to create library instruction that is relevant, effective, and interesting.

As with CAI, expert systems are effective for independent learners comfortable with computer technology. Expert systems are also highly transportable, because they can be made available on networks. Thus, an expert system can be shared by libraries. Library users can even acquire them for their own personal computers. Expert systems have the potential to be a strong delivery system for busy professionals who are geographically dispersed.

There are helpful articles on selecting expert system shells, multimedia, and hypertext software [74-75]. The Learning Center for Interactive Technology at the National Library of Medicine has a demonstration center for many of these types of programs, as well. The professional training literature can provide guidance in design for any computer-based training effort [76]. (For more information about computer-based programs, see Chapter 5.)

Summary

This chapter has described the wide range of educational programs and tools which health sciences librarians have available to meet the needs of their clientele. As librarians change the ways health information is organized and obtained, user education programs and materials will change as well. Expediting access to information in any format will redefine the content of educational programs.

Users who are increasingly eager to learn about, and use resources in, computerized formats have forced a rethinking of what constitutes effective teaching materials for user education. Through computer-based instructional formats, individuals are allowed a degree of self-direction that is unavailable even in private, guided sessions.

The wide array of delivery systems available makes it tempting to choose a medium that is interesting to the person designing the instruction without considering the target audience. For that reason, an instructional design process that makes choice of format dependent on variables such as goals and objectives helps assure a better educational product.

References

1. Allegri F. Maximizing resources: a look at library orientation programs. Med Ref Serv Q 1987 Summer;6(2):91-5.

2. Mitchell M, Saunders LM. The virtual library: an agenda for the 1990s. Comput Libr 1991 Apr;11(4):8-11.

3. Saunders LM. The virtual library today. Libr Admin Manage 1992 Spring;6(2):66-70.

4. Rice J, Jr. Strategies for library orientation. In: Rice J, Jr. Teaching library use: a guide for library instruction. Westport, CT: Greenwood, 1981:46-61.

5. Renford B, Hendrickson L. Orientation. In: Renford B, Hendrickson L. Bibliographic instruction: a handbook. New York, Neal-Schuman, 1980: 24-42.

6. Beaubien AK, Hogan SA, George MW. Planning a single lecture. In: Beaubien AK, Hogan SA, George MW. Learning the library: concepts and methods for effective bibliographic instruction. New York: R.R. Bowker, 1982:155-97.

7. Cimpl K. Clinical medical librarianship: a review of the literature. Bull Med Libr Assoc 1985 Jan;73(1):21-8.

8. Veentra RJ. A clinical librarian program in the intensive care unit. Crit Care Med 1992 Jul;20(7):1038-42.

9. Horak EB. Clinical librarianship in an era of end users. Med Ref Serv Q 1987 Summer;6(2):65-9.

10. Halsted DD, Ward DH, Neeley DM. The evolving role of clinical medical librarians. Bull Med Libr Assoc 1989 Jul;77(3):299-301.

11. Demas JM, Ludwig LT. Clinical medical librarian: the last unicorn? Bull Med Libr Assoc 1991 Jan;79(1):17-27.

12. Allegri F. One-on-one instruction. Med Ref Serv Q 1990 Summer;9(2):81-4.

13. Hardin Library for the Health Sciences. University of Iowa. Reference consultations. Information bulletin No. 25. Iowa City: Hardin Library for the Health Sciences, 1992.

14. Tooey MJ. Sharing our information expertise: a new role as consultants for health sciences librarians. Paper presented at the annual meeting of the Medical Library Association. Boston, MA: May 19-25, 1989.

15. Mularski CA, Bradigan PS. Library workshops for special audiences: secretaries, research assistants, and other support staff. Bull Med Libr Assoc 1988 Apr;76(2):151-4.

16. Brassil EC. Information management education: integrating the old with the new. Med Ref Serv Q 1985 Spring;4(1):91-5.

17. Wilson LA. Instruction as a reference service. In: Bopp RE, Smith LC, eds. Reference and information services: an introduction. Englewood, CO: Libraries Unlimited, 1991:124. (Library Science Text Series.)

18. Tooey MJ, Wester BR. Computer conferencing: a campus meets online. Online 1989 Jul;13(4):54-60.

19. Morgan EL. WAIS and gopher servers: a guide for librarian and Internet end-users. Westport, CT: Meckler, 1993.

20. Mikita EG, Drusedum LA. Introducing health sciences librarians to the Internet. Med Ref Serv Q 1993 Fall;12(3):1-12.

21. Tennant R, Ober J, Lipow AG. Crossing the Internet threshold: an instructional handbook. Berkeley, CA: Library Solutions Press, 1993:22,90.

22. Ibid., 24,98.

23. Buchanan HS, Fazzone N. Integrated information management and hospital libraries. Bull Med Libr Assoc 1985 Jan;73(1):47-54.

24. Graves KJ, Selig SA. Library instruction for medical students. Bull Med Libr Assoc 1986 Apr;74(2):126-30.

25. Moore M. Innovation and education: unlimited potential for the teaching library. Bull Med Libr Assoc 1989 Jan;77(1):26-32.

26. Burrows S, Ginn DS, Love N, Williams TL. A strategy for curriculum integration of information skills instruction. Bull Med Libr Assoc 1989 Jul;77(3):245-51.

27. Mueller MH, Foreman G. Library instruction for medical students during a curriculum elective. Bull Med Libr Assoc 1987 Jul;75(3):253-6.

28. Tooey MJ. Problem-based learning: getting started—part one. Med Ref Serv Q 1993 Fall;12(3):86-7.

29. Ibid., 85-9.

30. Rankin JA, ed. Highlighting problem-based learning and medical libraries. Bull Med Libr Assoc 1993 Jul;81(3):293-315.

31. Ibid.

32. Lunin LF, Ball MJ, eds. Perspectives on...information science and health informatics education. J Am Soc Info Sci 1989 Sep;40(5):364-77.

33. O'Leary M. Online clubs for micro users. Database 1988 Jun;11(3):122-4.

34. Hentz MB. Award winning online users groups. Online 1988 Jul;12(4):84-5.

35. Brown JF, Wood EH. Library-sponsored computer user groups. Bull Med Libr Assoc 1987 Apr;75(2):167-9.

36. Bearon LB, Hickman DH, Amara AH. Video journal club: combining video evaluation and continuing education. Gerontologist 1993 Jun;33(3):415-8.

37. Jones DA, Richmond CE, Christopher KA, Duggar DC. The journal club as an educational modality for librarians: the Louisiana State University Medical Center in Shreveport experience. LLA Bull 1993 Spring; 55(4):192-6.

38. Linzer M, Mercando A, Hupart KH. Role of a medical journal club in residency training. J Med Educ 1986 Jun; 61(6):471-3.

39. Jones, op.cit., 192.

40. Tibbles L, Sanford R. The research journal club: a mechanism for research utilization. Clin Nurse Spec 1994 Jan; 8(1):23-6.

41. Cooper JE. Using CAI to teach library skills. Coll Res Libr News 1993 Feb;54(2):78.

42. Zinn NW. Exhibits in health sciences libraries. Bull Med Libr Assoc 1984 Apr;72(2):193-7.

43. Schaeffer M. Library displays handbook. New York: H. W. Wilson, 1991.

44. Johnson C. Signs of the times: signage in the library. Wilson Libr Bull 1993 Nov;68(3):40-2.

45. Van Allen PR. A good library sign system: is it possible? Ref Serv Rev 1984 Summer;12(2):102-6.

46. Mallery MS, DeVore RE. A sign system for libraries. Chicago: American Library Association, 1982.

47. Pollet D. You can get there from here: new directions in library signage. Wilson Libr Bull 1976 Feb;50(6):456-62.

48. Kosmin LJ. The electronic reference desk: platform for library newsletter (presented at CIL Conference '91). Libr Soft Rev 1991 Jul/Aug;10(4):278-9.

49. Russo-Martin E, Grefsheim SF. How to publish a library newsletter. Med Ref Serv Q 1984 Winter;3(4):27-34.

50. Ford S. The library newsletter: is it for you? Coll Res Libr News 1988 Nov;49(10):678-82.

51. Hooker F. Public relations the old-fashioned way: newsletters. Wilson Libr Bull 1986 Feb; 60(6):22-6.

52. Beaubien AK, Hogan SA, George MW. Learning the library: concepts and methods for effective bibliographic instruction. New York: R.R. Bowker, 1982:48,51.

53. Cipolla KG. M.I.T.'s point-of-use concept: a five-year update. J Acad Libr 1980 Jan;5(6):326-8.

54. Canfield MP. Library pathfinders. Drexel Libr Q 1972 Jul;8(3):287-300.

55. Fink D. Process and politics in library research: a model for course design. Chicago: American Library Association, 1989:9-11.

56. Freedman JL, Bantly HA, comp. Information searching: a handbook for designing and creating instructional programs. Rev. ed. Metuchen, NJ: Scarecrow, 1982:26-65.

57. Weiner DJ. The video source book. 15th ed. Detroit: Gale Research, 1994.

58. Van Nostran WJ. Scriptwriter's handbook. White Plains, NY: Knowledge Industry, 1989.

59. McNally T. Creative approaches to video for bibliographic instruction. Chicago: Association of College and Research Libraries, American Library Association, 1985. (ACRL CE-206 Continuing Education Program.)

60. Shedlock J, Tawyea EW. Library orientation on videotape: production planning and administrative support. Med Ref Serv Q 1989 Summer;8(2):15-24.

61. Turner A. Computer-assisted instruction in academic libraries (12 situational characteristics that seem to favor CAI applications). J Acad Libr 1990 Jan;15(6):352-4.

62. Steinberg ER. Teaching computers to teach. 2d ed. Hillsdale, NJ: Lawrence Erlbaum Associates, 1991.

63. Cooper, op. cit., 75-8.

64. Bellamy LM, Silver JT, Selig SA, Givens MK. Linking information about the library to the library user through hypermedia. In: Kingsland LC, ed. Proceedings of the thirteenth annual symposium on computer applications in medical care. Washington, DC: IEEE Computer Society, 1989:853-7.

65. Bailey CW, Jr. Intelligent multimedia computer systems: emerging information resources in the network environment. Libr Hi Tech 1990;8(1):29.

66. D'Ignazio F. Getting a jump on the future: everything you'll ever need to know about multimedia authoring tools. Electronic Learning 1992 Nov/Dec;12(3):28,30-1.

67. Stewart S. Interactive healthcare directory. Alexandria, VA: Stewart, 1992.

68. Slice of Life VI (videodisc). Salt Lake City: University of Utah School of Medicine, 1992.

69. Rogers EM. Diffusion of innovation. New York: Macmillan, 1983.

70. Orwig G, Barron A. Expert systems: an overview for teacher-librarians. Emer Libr 1992 Jan/Feb;19(3):19-21.

71. Gunning K. The intelligent reference information system: the effect on public services of implementing a CD-ROM LAN and expert system. Libr Admin Manage 1992 Summer;6(3):146-53.

72. Riggs DE. Productivity increases in public services: are expert systems the answer? J Libr Admin 1988;9(4):93-4.

73. Binkley RD, Parrott JR. A reference-librarian model for computer-aided library instruction. Info Serv Use 1987;7(1):31-8.

74. Quinn K. Expert system shells: what to look for. Ref Serv Rev 1990 Spring;18(1):83-6.

75. Tolhurst D. A checklist for evaluating content-based hypertext computer software. Educ Tech 1992 Mar;32(3):17-21.

76. Fitz J. Conquering the dreaded electronic textbook. Training 1990 May (suppl);27(5):15,17-9.

may be a familiar one. Marketing has applications well beyond the for-profit setting: part of it is concerned with advertising a commodity after determining the product needs of potential customers. The commodity, in this case, is educational services. The means for obtaining these services may or may not involve the exchange of money. The potential customers, for the most part, are health professionals, students, and staff [1-2].

An analogy with the commercial world is apt. Manufacturers advertise products and services of which consumers are not yet aware. In the library setting, the products are new or better information sources and services, assistance, or classes. A consumer may learn from a magazine advertisement that a certain toothpaste claims to fight cavities better, but do nurses see posters in the library that tell them which index covers more nursing journals than another?

Users may not think of the librarian as a teacher. It may not occur to a group of physical therapists that a class could be organized to help them with their special needs. The library must promote its teaching role—the idea that librarians are willing and able to share their skills through organized classes and courses [3-4].

Marketing is frequently confused with promotion, public relations, and even selling. In more accurate terms, marketing has been described as a five-part, cyclical process. The five parts are

1. Market segmentation.
2. Market positioning.
3. Consumer analysis.
4. Marketing program.
5. Marketing audit [5].

These can be translated in the library context into information gathering about library users, ranking groups of users and services, determining user needs, planning and promoting a coordinated program, and evaluating the program. This final step, evaluation, leads back to information gathering and a repeat of the process.

It is not the intent here to give detailed instructions on how marketing is to be conducted. What follows is a brief outline of the process combined with examples from the user education perspective. Emphasis has been given to needs assessment and promotion, about which many questions arise.

Information Gathering (Market Segmentation)

Various strategies can be used to find out who are the actual and potential users of educational services. It is also important to find out who will remain nonusers despite marketing efforts. Those who have other sources for training could be part of this last group.

> Market segmentation is a way of acknowledging that libraries cannot be all things to all people...Market segmentation provides focus and helps us to set priorities. If it is practiced effectively, it ensures greater responsiveness to the needs of specific user groups [6].

Actual and potential users can be determined by keeping statistics on program participants and those who ask reference questions that result in instruction. Other sources of data include

> ...circulation and reference statistics, complaints and compliments from the suggestion box, planning documents, the library's mission statement, analyses of special programs and services, and staff observations [7].

Other data can be obtained from persons offering similar or related instruction within or near the parent institution. For example, the number and type of staff within the hospital who are attending classes broadcast by satellite might prove useful. All of these numbers must then be related to the totals available from the personnel department, annual reports, and other sources. Demographic and geographic information should be added, as available. The result will be a chart of the proportions of users who are actual, potential, and nonuser.

Ranking Users and Services (Market Positioning)

"Market targeting is evaluating each [market] segment's attractiveness and selecting one or more of the market segments to enter" [8]. Because there are many potential market segments, a library must limit the number it chooses to pursue. The library may also choose to go after markets sequentially to avoid large outlays of resources. A library

> ...must select target markets that provide the best opportunity, that most clearly seem to need its product, and that can most efficiently and cost-effectively be reached through standard promotional and

> advertising methods. In effect, the company [library] must select a target market that will give the highest return on the marketing investment [9].

If none exist, policy statements need to be developed to determine how to provide instruction most effectively to help the largest number of people in the primary user groups. These policy decisions are based on the mission and goals of the library and the parent organization.

Determining User Needs (Consumer Analysis)

As part of marketing library services to users, it is helpful to assess how most users look for information when they come to the library. Information-seeking behaviors are related here to the educational and instructional needs of users. This is commonly referred to as doing a needs assessment.

Librarians may naively assume that library users will approach information sources in the way librarians would. Users will use subject headings, go to the appropriate indexes, search the literature exhaustively, scan new books regularly, and keep their own files in immaculate order—organized by Medical Subject Headings (MeSH) terms, of course! Interviews with users often tell a different tale of serendipitous browsing among the recent journal issues, online searching for *breast cancer* or *heart attack* (rather than the thesaurus terms, BREAST NEOPLASMS or MYOCARDIAL INFARCTION), judging books by their titles alone, and handing annotated search retrieval to a secretary with the request to, "Get these articles from the library and file them."

A systematic study of users' performance in finding the information they need may indicate the effectiveness of education programs [10-11]. The library may have the materials users are looking for, but the users are unable to find them. A study of these situations may indicate needs that cross a variety of disciplines and types of users. Using subject headings, recognizing the difference between a citation to a journal and to a book chapter, understanding medical terminology, using basic online search techniques—these are examples of instructional topics that may be needed by many different groups.

Both random and systematic observation of users looking for information will provide clues about their information-seeking needs. Some ideas for informal data gathering are

- Putting up signs encouraging users to ask for help.
- Educating staff to accept complaints in nondefensive ways and gather information from users.

- Asking users if they found what they were looking for.
- Asking users if they are familiar with, or need help with, an index or computer system.
- Asking users for their recommendations on improving signs and written instructions.

A more systematic way of collecting such information is the survey. Design and implementation are covered in the literature [12-13]. Questionnaires about needs can be distributed in a variety of ways, some more assertive than others. The most passive method is to leave questionnaires by the catalog and checkout counter. The response rate may be increased by handing the forms to users entering or leaving the library or a service area. A verbal incentive is recommended: "We're interested in whether you found what you were looking for. Would you answer a few questions?" (For more information about data collection, see Chaper 5.)

To gather information about users and how they can be helped, librarians need to take an active role [14]. Some library users know they need help, but may not know whether they can obtain it. Others are unaware that they are not using what is available to their best advantage. Still others are intimidated and afraid to ask [15]. While these problems can and do apply to any age group, users who did not grow up with computer technology may be in need of special help with new automated systems. The installation of online resources may alarm them, but they are embarrassed to ask for assistance. Other users see innovations as an opportunity to approach and ask the librarian.

Librarians may determine that an entire department is having difficulty finding material on a subject; the need for group training is obvious. Faculty may give library assignments without awareness of the stress placed on students and library resources. These situations pose a particular challenge. If approached tactfully and in a spirit of cooperation, these faculty may welcome assistance in improving library assignments. While one-on-one help at the catalog or reference desk will aid individuals with their immediate needs, group instruction usually makes more efficient use of resources and is less threatening to users who are hesitant to ask for help.

The following examples show how librarians can learn, by observation and interviews, what kinds of instructional programs users need. Many other examples exist in the literature [16-18].

Example: Like busy clinicians and researchers, some faculty will send others to the library on their behalf and some never seem to need the library at all. Every library has regulars who know librarians by name and clearly understand how to find information efficiently. These faculty may be willing to come to a panel session or librarians' meeting where they will describe their own and their colleagues' habits and needs. They may also have suggestions as to why their colleagues do not come to the library or have difficulty using it.

Example: Laboratory and office personnel are populations that are sometimes overlooked by librarians. These staff members are frequently used by other health professionals to locate library materials [19-20]. Clerical and research assistants may have other motives for wanting to know how to use the library effectively—to do a good job for the boss and avoid returning to the office empty-handed. Many a reference librarian has noticed that the same laboratory technician comes regularly to the library with some barely legible scribbling on a piece of paper. A good deal of the citation may be missing or erroneous. No one has explained the differences among various citation formats. The jobs of the technician and the secretary would become easier if they received instruction on finding materials in the library.

Example: Library staff may observe a physician or student fruitlessly searching *breast cancer.* Some library users may not be aware that many subject catalogs and online systems use controlled vocabularies. Researchers may be very annoyed when their own articles on a subject do not seem to be in the bibliographic database; instruction in performing an author search may solve the problem.

These examples have been given in detail to demystify the needs assessment process.

Planning a Coordinated Program (Marketing Program)

Once user groups and users' needs have been identified, a coordinated plan can be drawn up. The result of this step is a customized plan for the prime mix of products and services, price and cost, location and method of delivery, and promotion of the products and services [21].

The promotion part of this marketing step can trace any number of paths. The means selected will depend on the results of completing the previous marketing steps. Some examples of promotion techniques follow.

Example: Academic librarians with faculty status or the equivalent may have the opportunity to sit on curriculum committees. Self-evaluation study groups or curriculum review committees may also include librarians. Involvement in other groups can foster relationships which promote the inclusion of the library in decision-making bodies such as advisory boards or staff assemblies. These all offer opportunities to promote the teaching role of the library, as well as specific programs.

Example: Publishing compelling statistics and evaluations in library or other newsletters, or making them known at clinical department or faculty meetings, can help increase library involvement in staff development or the curriculum. Those in positions of authority can be made aware of how many of their employees or students have attended library education programs and what they should be able to do as a result of the instruction. Publishing library statistics, selectively and attractively, can promote services to those who are otherwise unaware that the library is anything more than a collection of printed materials.

Many potential users do not come to the library because they are unaware that it contains information they need or because they do not know how to find the information. The library can reach this population through instruction. Some suggestions for making nonusers aware of the library's existence and services are

- Contact departments to offer tailor-made education programs; these offers can be made at department meetings or in the library's or the target population's newsletter [22].
- Ask the administrator or personnel director about being part of established orientation programs.
- Be on mailing lists to find out when new groups arrive.
- Ask to be invited to attend meetings, orientations, and welcome parties and discuss the library's educational services informally with other attendees.
- Post announcements and class schedules in strategic locations.
- Visit departments, clinics, offices, and labs.
- Send mailings tailored to particular groups and individuals.
- Set up pilot classes tailored to specific groups to determine interest as well as to promote educational services.

If the busy clinician can be persuaded, in advance, that his staff will do a better job at the library after training, the librarian's task is much easier. Grateful staff who have been helped by the librarian can be encouraged to go back to the office and suggest training for others. Supervisors may never have been in the library themselves and may have little idea what is involved in finding the proceedings of a meeting, an article written sometime during the last decade, or a book chapter with its own authors and no reference to the overall title. If these supervisors can be reached, either directly or through the employees they send to the library, everyone will be served better.

New is regarded by advertising professionals as an eye-catching word. When the library does something new, it should be advertised. Examples of changes that deserve attention are listed below. These are all opportunities to offer education and training in the use of new products and offer refreshers on the use of traditional resources.

- Closing the card catalog.
- Shifts in the collection.
- Acquiring the first or additional CD-ROMs.
- A new online vendor.
- Upgrades to hardware.
- New software.
- Adding telefacsimile (FAX) service.
- GRATEFUL MED updates.
- New staff.
- New staff expertise or training.
- New users ("Welcome New Residents!").

Suggestions for promoting these events include putting up signs, announcing events in newsletters, posting notes on electronic bulletin boards, contacting key individuals, stuffing mailboxes, and pinning notices to bulletin boards. If the change is major, the library can put up balloons, offer refreshments, or have an open house. *Marketing Treasures,* a newsletter aimed at libraries, contains many more promotion ideas, as well as articles on all aspects of marketing.

Evaluating the Program (Marketing Audit)

Chapter 5, Evaluation and Future Trends, provides complete and detailed information on educational program evaluation techniques. Zachert and Williams provide a very thought-provoking and practical discussion of quantitative measures of marketing programs [23].

Staffing and Staff Development

In the past, user education was handled primarily in the library, solely by the library, and using only library resources. Librarians taught users to identify materials in card catalogs that the librarians themselves created; they helped users understand indexes that librarians had been familiar with for all of their careers; they explained call numbers, main entries, corporate authors, key words in context, and the mysteries of citation indexing. Librarians involved in user education had to learn basic teaching techniques, but the subject matter posed few problems because it was already so familiar.

In the workplace of today, librarians may be working with computer departments, institutional information management divisions, or external consultants. Since no one could have predicted the changes of the past decade, no systematic training or retraining was envisioned. Now, in addition to learning how to teach, technological developments require that staff be continually updated on the latest changes so that they have the expertise to help users [24].

Improving staff expertise in both teaching and technology takes money, time, and intellectual energy. Existing staff may need retraining and new staff may be needed who have the skills necessary for teaching in a technologically advanced environment. Innovation can be stressful, and some staff may resist new techniques and argue against the need to teach them to users. Managing staff in this era of technological change requires psychological energy on the part of supervisors, who may need to sell new ideas as well as teach them to staff.

In some situations, a library may be able to replace or hire staff who will have teaching responsibilities; at other times, existing staff may be offered the opportunity to move into these areas and be trained, as necessary. The following section discusses options for staffing teaching programs. Administrative structures, recruitment, hiring, development, quality control, and the rewards unique to educational services are included.

Administrative Structures

Most health sciences libraries include educational services as a part of public services. In larger libraries, responsibility for education is either given to the reference department or to a separate user education department. However, the model of an academic library with a bibliographic instruction librarian, or an education department, is, by no means, the only way of helping users become information literate. Some other configurations are described below.

- One librarian delivers all educational services and all other library services. The librarian may arrange for others from outside the library to teach, e.g., systems analysts, database consultants, other librarians.
- All librarians share the teaching load.
- All reference librarians share the teaching load.
- A user education coordinator plans and organizes instruction, but other librarians share the teaching load. The coordinator usually works in the reference department.
- A user education librarian has sole responsibility for teaching. This librarian could report to a department head, typically in public services, or could head a separate department with additional educational librarians or support staff.
- A user education staff is coordinated by the head of another department.
- A user education librarian, reporting to the library director, has responsibility and authority to contract with other library departments for class development and teaching.
- Leadership for educational services resides in the library, but instructors are recruited primarily from outside the library.
- Educational services is an umbrella department, encompassing such areas as reference, database searching, consultation, and microcomputers [25-27].

In some settings, the teaching is done through a learning resources center. The center may or may not be part of the library. The center's staff may be librarians or computer experts. Librarians and computer consultants may collaborate in teaching. Classes using computers for literature searching or file management may be included on a roster with basic microcomputing, word processing, or database management. Advantages are that the librarians will gain in computer expertise and the consultants will learn more about library operations and the needs of library users [28].

In any setting in which several people are involved in teaching, one person needs to coordinate the program. The coordinator makes sure that the syllabus is interpreted in the same way by every teacher and holds regular meetings so that all the teachers can share experiences and discuss improvements. Ideally, a user should receive the same information, presented in a similar fashion, regardless of which librarian is teaching. It is important that within any library the teaching program is consistent in content and quality.

A coordinator also arranges the calendar, makes sure that appropriate records are kept, and collects any evaluation forms or other data that help ensure quality. The librarian who acts as coordinator need not be in a supervisory or management position. A reference section, for example, may assign responsibilities so that one librarian coordinates search services while another coordinates user education. Yet, all the librarians in the section do both searching and teaching.

Teaching can be shared in several ways: by alternating a class among teachers, by team teaching, or by specializing in particular subjects. Class preparation can also be a team effort—tasks such as research, writing, collecting samples or examples, and designing audiovisual aids can be done by different people.

Many factors must be considered in organizing staff to provide educational services. Some of these are user demand, number of staff, goals and scope of instruction, willingness and skills of librarians, and the visibility and priority desired for the library's educational role.

Educational programs are certainly not unique to health sciences libraries. Organizations outside the field may be consulted for valuable insights in all areas of instruction, including administrative structures. (For a list of relevant organizations, see Appendices A and B.)

Types of Personnel Involved

The three primary categories of personnel involved in user education are librarians, support staff, and nonlibrary staff. In today's health sciences libraries, public services librarians have the major responsibility for teaching users. Excellent communication skills have always been desirable in candidates for public services positions and reference work has, for some time, involved elements of teaching. Since public services librarians are usually trained to relate well to users, they have been chosen for teaching assignments.

Over the years, there has been increased participation in offering educational programs by library staff other than those in public services. Technical services librarians and support staff and microcomputer or learning resources staff have had roles that range from teaching to designing audiovisual materials. Seeking this help and then providing the coordination and training needed are crucial for seamless educational presentations.

In larger settings, librarians may be supported by clerical or support staff who help with the scheduling and advertising, preparation of written materials, and equipment [29]. Support staff may also help conduct tours and orientations or provide basic instruction on using the online catalog. The larger the teaching program, the more support staff are needed.

The impact of computerization has been evident in the presence of nonlibrary personnel in user education programs. This is most obvious in the collaboration between libraries and microcomputer or mainframe computer departments. Computer consultants and others may teach in or support the educational services of the library.

Professionals

Professional librarians do the bulk of planning, managing, class preparation, and teaching for user education. Although public services librarians usually perform these functions, technical services, learning resources, and computer services librarians are playing an increasingly significant role in user education.

Relationships between technical and public services personnel have changed with the advent of the online catalog. As remote access to online catalogs became possible, user populations grew and diversified. Menu design, screen presentation, and online documentation have been changed to aid these new users. User education staff in public service areas need to interact closely with computer departments as well as technical services. As an example, interface design discussions should include the designers as well as the librarians who are going to be explaining the menus to users. Class evaluations and users' comments should be used as feedback to improve existing interfaces and construct new ones. User education librarians are ideally suited for helping with online documentation and suggesting terms or instructions that users will understand. Technical services staff have thorough knowledge of the collection and its arrangement, as well as automated systems, so they are invaluable partners in education. If they also enjoy teaching, they can be included in the education program in additional ways. This is true of both librarians and support staff.

In cases where the library has its own computer consultants on staff, the consultants may teach classes. A typical division of labor might be that consultants teach basic computer literacy, word processing, using electronic mail and telecommunications software, and setting up networks; while librarians teach database searching, indexing and reprint file management, research techniques, and bibliography compilation.

Support Staff

These personnel can assist in a variety of ways, depending on their willingness, training, and the time constraints of their existing duties. Support staff can conduct orientations or tours. They can teach users to locate materials in the online catalog or to understand the arrangement of the stacks. Other examples of help they can provide include printing and distributing class rosters, keeping registration lists, reminding participants that class is coming up, collecting fees, entering participant or evaluation data into a database, setting up the classroom, printing and collating handouts, and filing class materials.

A particularly useful role for support staff is to assist in teaching nonhomogeneous groups of attendees. A class that includes students, secretaries, clinicians, and hospital volunteers is more difficult to teach than one where the members of the group have similar responsibilities and experience. A slow learner, a person who asks many questions, or someone hampered by language differences can slow down the class and make teaching a challenge. A way to expedite the class is to position another staff member in the room, either behind the computer screens watching what students are typing, or walking around the room making sure everyone is following in the index or text. This assistant can help answer questions from students. If support staff are familiar with computers, they can also supervise hands-on sessions or provide assistance with hardware and software.

Nonlibrary Staff

Outside teachers may be invited to be part of the library's educational program. For example, staff with more extensive computer expertise may be borrowed from institutional computer departments. Vendors may be invited to demonstrate search techniques. They may provide instruction for a fee or free; some require a guaranteed audience.

Library users may like to know more about genetic databases, resume writing, medical terminology, data analysis, biostatistics, or medical jurisprudence. The library may invite professionals from these disciplines to be part of the teaching schedule. Library users with special expertise can become instructors, as well.

In a very small library, bringing in other staff or users to teach may be the only way the librarian can offer classes. In a decade when all institutional units are struggling to justify their existence, interdepartmental cooperation and an increased perception of the role of the library will benefit all.

Regardless of the types of personnel involved, program coordination becomes increasingly important when classes vary widely in type, subject matter, and teaching staff. Rather than a hodgepodge of unrelated sessions, the program should appear as a seamless whole, with logical connections to library operations. Classes should be publicized so that they are tied together for maximum benefit to the user. Basic computer literacy, for example, could be suggested as a prerequisite for database searching;

reprint file management could be a logical follow-up to downloading search retrieval.

All library staff need to know what user education is offered, whom to contact to arrange it, what categories of library users are eligible for what kinds of classes, and what prerequisites and fees exist. If, for example, only library card holders can sign up for MEDLINE classes, both the access services staff who give out cards and the reference staff who teach MEDLINE need to understand this. If users want document delivery from the MEDLINE searches they have been trained to perform themselves, everyone involved in document delivery—photocopy services, interlibrary loan, FAX machine operators—needs to understand the process of searching, checking the library's own holdings, and passing requests on to interlibrary loan. It may be helpful for those who are not teaching to attend a user education class. This would give them a better understanding of what user education is all about, promote a feeling of participation, and enable them to answer questions more comfortably.

Recruiting and Hiring

It may not be necessary to recruit teachers if existing staff are already willing and capable teachers. Librarians on staff may have the background that is needed but have never been asked if they would like to perform these duties. An atmosphere needs to be created that encourages these staff to volunteer. If all library staff are expected to teach, this obligation must be reflected in the recruitment, orientation, and continuing education of new personnel [30]. Library staff may have an interest in teaching and would gladly accept training if it is offered. Administrators and education coordinators need to examine their preconceptions about what makes someone a good teacher before looking beyond their own personnel [31].

The advantages of using existing staff are that they know the user population, they understand library policies, and they are already on the payroll. Teaching may add an interesting and rewarding dimension to their jobs and can expand career options. However, if other responsibilities are not reallocated, existing staff may not have the time to add teaching responsibilities to their duties. Teaching may be more time-consuming than anyone anticipated or staff may not be as good at teaching as was hoped.

Teachers recruited from outside the library can be evaluated more critically through a formal interview process. They may bring fresh ideas and teach staff, as well as users. Obviously, candidates for library instructors may be found by including teaching experience in a job announcement and looking for the necessary skills in the resumes of those who apply. Other recruiting techniques include the following:

- Contacting education departments or user education coordinators of other libraries, both health sciences and others.
- Advertising in the newsletters of appropriate organizations. (For a selective list of these, see Appendix B.)
- Contacting possible candidates who teach in the institution's computer services department.

The types of experience and skills a candidate would need will vary according to the library's goals and programs. Working knowledge of specific resources and systems may be required. For example, two years online searching experience on MEDLARS or BRS may be a minimum requirement. A list of instructional knowledge and skills to look for in applicants includes

> ...an understanding of and expertise in learning theory and cognitive psychology, curriculum and instructional development, instructional systems design, educational needs assessment and analysis, learning style appraisal, instructional methodologies, and evaluation of learning outcomes [32].

The *College & Research Libraries News, MLA News,* and the Library Orientation/instruction EXchange (LOEX) newsletter job advertisements can be checked for ideas on how to translate this list into practical terms for recruiting.

Once applicants have been selected for interviews, there are some steps that apply specifically to user education. At a minimum, interviewees should be asked to make an oral presentation to all library staff, or a select group of users, on a user education topic. Samples of syllabi or other course materials they have produced should be requested in advance of an interview. Other steps might include contacting people who have attended programs the applicants have offered.

It is still rare to find applicants who possess all of the desired attributes listed here. In any case, the library administration needs to be committed to developing teaching staff along these lines.

Once an instructional librarian has been hired, it is important that the library director or immediate supervisor introduce the librarian to the deans, department heads, and key personnel of appropriate user groups. This is especially critical in larger settings in which a coordinator or head of educational services is hired. This step is not only politically wise, but it is another opportunity to promote educational services.

Developing Educational Services Staff

It is a fragile assumption that almost any librarian is willing or able to teach. If a library is new to formal teaching or has a number of new staff who are unfamiliar with teaching, there are some questions that should be asked. Not every librarian makes a good teacher. It may not even be necessary that everyone learn how to teach. Some staff may be unwilling instructors and may never develop the desire or ability to teach. It would be better to look elsewhere.

That said, sometimes there are existing staff who can be tapped for teaching roles. Both librarians and support staff from departments other than public services may be excellent teachers. Microcomputer technicians, systems analysts, or other computer professionals and support staff can be significant members of the teaching program. While some may be superb teachers, some may need to be coached so that their audiences are not overwhelmed with technical jargon and unnecessary behind-the-scenes complexities.

Problems first-time teachers may experience include nervousness, lack of organization, a tendency to ramble, speaking too slowly or too quickly, too intimidating an approach, a cold or impersonal demeanor, lack of confidence, or an apologetic attitude.

Areas for Development

Instructors will benefit from some background reading or even course work in adult learning or teaching methods. Competencies are described in the literature [33-36]. (For more information on topics for staff development, see Chapter 2.) Library staff must also be committed to learning new technologies. Existing staff may develop their skills over the years and learn gradually as technologies are introduced, but new staff may have to become computer literate and learn to use the online catalog, CD-ROM, electronic databases, e-mail, and FAX—all as part of initial training [37].

Computer literacy may include word processing, database management, and online systems. Familiarity with CD-ROM and the ability to compare that technology with dial-up access or locally mounted databases are desirable skills. This list can be expanded to information literacy—a concept well-defined by the American Library Association. Information literacy also includes search strategy construction, familiarity with key information sources, and evaluation and effective use of information [38-39]. It is assumed that librarians are already information literate when they take on a role in educational services. Continued development in this area is vital [40].

Another important teaching skill is the ability to write handouts and other documentation. Librarians whose prior training has not included teaching methods, educational psychology, or instructional design may need help in crafting documentation. Those without artistic ability may need to call upon colleagues for help with signs and layout. (For further information on creating documentation and signage, see Chapter 3.)

Methods for Training Staff

Both professional and support staff have become better teachers and computer literate by various means. These can be summarized as

- Reading and self-instruction.
- In-house training by colleagues or institutional staff.
- Trial and error out of personal interest.
- Requesting hardware and software on a trial basis.
- Formal continuing education.
  Locally by professional organizations.
  At national meetings.
  From outside vendors.

Some techniques for making teachers feel more comfortable in front of groups include

- Extending components of the reference interview and one-on-one help to teaching in small groups and then larger classes.
- Rehearsing in front of colleagues (also a quality control technique).
- Starting out as an assistant to another teacher.
- Beginning with small groups (two or three people) or groups that have proven friendly in the past.
- Having an approachable colleague critique the class.
- Following a highly structured syllabus.
- Receiving coaching that confidence grows with experience.
- Participating in evaluations of classes.
- Holding meetings to share experiences and go over evaluations.
- Attending classes on teaching techniques or public speaking.

An in-house training program can be started gradually by individuals sharing tips and techniques. At some point, a meeting or class can be held regularly to keep everyone at the same level of knowledge and competence. A larger library may bring in employees from other divisions of the institution or hire experts to present seminars [41].

Continuing education programs on bibliographic instruction, microcomputers, and database searching have been developed by organizations such as the Medical Library Association [42] and many of its local chapters. Commercial vendors offer conferences such as Meckler's "Computers in Libraries" and the "ONLINE/CD-ROM" meeting from Online, Inc. Details about these conferences are published in the sponsors' corresponding journals, *Computers in Libraries* and *Online.* These are also titles many librarians read to stay abreast of developments. An electronic discussion list, Public-Access Computer Systems (PACS-L), is available on Internet and there is an electronic newletter of the same name. (See Appendix C.) The related print journal is *The Public-Access Computer Systems Review.*

Journals in the health sciences that routinely carry articles about user education and reviews of software include the *Bulletin of the Medical Library Association* and *Medical Reference Services Quarterly.* Other titles that publish useful information for staff development and training include *Database, CD-ROM Professional, Reference Services Review, Library Software Review,* and the publications of the Library and Information Technology Association (LITA).

Formal courses are one of several options for developing user education staff. If the idea of standing up in front of a group is psychologically intimidating, training and management consultant firms offer classes on making effective presentations. There are also speech clubs, such as Toastmasters International. It has chapters across the country and can be a fun, nonthreatening forum for practice and feedback. Local universities, community colleges, and public libraries can assist the interested person in finding these types of continuing education opportunities.

Library professional organizations occasionally offer workshops, video courses, and other forms of instruction on communication skills. (See Appendix A.) In addition, all of the groups listed in Appendix B provide continuing education programs and materials specific to user education.

Learning and teaching are closely linked. Librarians may learn by teaching one another before teaching users. Anyone who teaches and has not had formal teacher training can benefit from a train-the-trainer program that discusses the basic principles of adult learning theory and practice. Support staff who help users directly need to be trained along with librarians.

Time must be set aside for systematic training, as well as for attending professional meetings and reading the literature. Staff development is an ongoing endeavor. Just as hardware and software are being constantly improved and upgraded, so librarians must improve their skills and adapt to new technologies and new teaching methods as they arise.

The past decade has seen the proliferation of books, articles, continuing education programs, professional meeting presentations, and personal communications that have helped library staff to become computer literate and more knowledgeable instructors.

The personal communications mentioned cannot be overemphasized as a means of staff development. These communications include correspondence, telephone, and electronic mail (e-mail). Many libraries, and the Medical Library Association, now provide access to various academic, commercial, and government networks that allow Internet or BITNET connections. A librarian who participates in an e-mail forum can throw out a question one day and receive dozens of replies from all over the country, if not the world, by tomorrow. One such forum is devoted to medical libraries and another to library instruction. (See Appendix C.) An example of an actual question that generated some weeks of discussion was whether students who had received instruction in using subject headings were observed using them after class. Librarians who reported that students continued to use title words with inappropriate Boolean operators tended to argue that instruction in subject headings was a waste of time; others insisted that the training must be done properly in order to have an effect on student behavior. Clearly, the use of these discussion forums can be valuable as well as time-consuming; librarians must be cautious in deciding how much time to devote to them.

Quality Control

Even though personalities and teaching styles vary, a user education coordinator should ensure that curriculum content, teaching goals, and handouts are of high quality. There are a number of ways to achieve consistency and quality control.

Curriculum Review

The most effective curriculum review is conducted by a team. This team could be simply the proposed teacher and a supervisor or the teacher and a trial group of students. Or the team may be the reference section, the learning resources section, all librarians involved in teaching, or the rest of the library staff. This review process ensures that curricula do not conflict or overlap unnecessarily and that content is accurate and consistent with library policies. An additional benefit is that users or librarians, other than the teacher, know what is being taught and can encourage appropriate users to attend. Some classes, such as database searching, may be taught by several librarians. Other classes, such as electronic mail or reprint filing, may be the particular specialty of one or two staff members. Curriculum review ensures consistency from teacher to teacher and confirms that these classes are appropriate to the program as a whole.

Practice Sessions

New classes are presented to a group of peers as a rehearsal or dry run. Classes are not taught to users until the review group deems them ready. This kind of peer review can be more intimidating than actually teaching users. If the size of the library does not permit this kind of review, selected users can be asked to evaluate a proposed new class or training session. However, constructive criticism from peers can be an invaluable learning experience [43].

An aid to peer review is videotaping the practice session and playing it back to the teacher or the group. Having an expert critique the videotape with the instructor is extremely helpful. This technology can also be used for self-evaluation [44]. Videotaping in this manner is common in the business world but can be emotionally difficult to experience. However, when done well, it results in more confident, polished, and effective teachers. Recording the learners' reactions and involvement in the instruction is a vital part of this technique [45]. The availability of home video equipment makes this a feasible method in the smallest settings. Another option is to invite a colleague to sit in on sessions to critique them.

Editing Documentation

If many teachers use the same syllabus, it should reflect the organization and content everyone will use, and instructors should collaborate and agree on the design and substance. An overall editor is needed to ensure consistency. Class materials should be reviewed and revised regularly, not only to ensure currency, but to remove material that is less successful and to reinforce ideas that work well. Handouts, syllabi, teaching aids, and evaluation forms can be reviewed and edited by the same person or group.

The style of documents should conform to a predetermined library standard and documents should be given standardized file names and stored together. With word processing, this is an easy task. Handling documentation is discussed more fully under support issues. As with curricula and teaching methods, the goal here is consistent quality.

Reward Mechanisms

There are a number of rewards that are unique to those involved in educational services. Librarians developing courses may be given time off from other duties, perhaps working at home or away from the office hubbub. A one-day planning retreat off-site for those involved in teaching can be arranged, with refreshments provided by the library or administrative unit. Librarians from other local libraries can be invited for a discussion over breakfast or lunch, funded in the same way. Minisabbaticals may be offered, to be used however the librarian instructor sees fit. These can be for lengths of a day, a week or a series of half-days. Besides more general library meetings, teachers may be sent to special conferences such as LOEX or the Symposium on Computer Applications in Medical Care (SCAMC). Team teaching a class that is normally taught solo can be fun and entertaining, besides reinforcing relationships between colleagues.

Teaching has its own rewards, as well. Course development and teaching successes can be beneficial additions to a resume or promotion dossier. Teaching brings librarians into contact with clinicians, faculty, and students in a situation where the roles are different; the librarian is seen as an expert and a mentor. In some settings, educational services are viewed as new, special, or esteemed, and sharing this limelight is refreshing. Finally, teaching can strengthen self-confidence and bring out new aspects of one's personality.

Support Issues

Documentation

Many different types of documentation are needed for user education. These include signs, information sheets, registration forms, syllabi and handouts, cheat sheets, evaluations, and office statistics [46].

If someone in the library is particularly good at freehand drawing or photography, these talents can be put to good use in designing professional-looking, interesting teaching materials. However, most of these materials need not be created from scratch. Help can be obtained from a number of sources. Other librarians are pleased to share their materials; they may be contacted individually, or through clearinghouses established by professional organizations. The library literature will lead to librarians who have established programs and are willing to share ideas and materials. Some journals, such as *Medical Reference Services Quarterly*, have columns devoted to user education. The Association of College and Research Libraries (ACRL) has a very active Bibliographic Instruction Section. The American Library Association also has a Library Instruction Round Table. Another source of ideas is LOEX—an exchange system to which libraries may subscribe to borrow materials; LOEX also holds conferences at which materials are displayed. The Public Services Section (PSS) of the Medical Library Association also has an exchange program for borrowing materials developed by other libraries. The exchange is managed by the PSS General Reference Special Interest Group (SIG). Lists of available exchange materials are printed in the Section's newsletter. Sometimes materials are available for loan or purchase. MLA may be contacted for the current SIG coordinator and newsletter editor. (For a list of addresses, see Appendix B.) In any case, the producer should be acknowledged if any part of a handout, chart, transparency, or text is used by another library.

In a setting where many librarians are teaching a variety of classes, it is more efficient and frugal to keep indexed files of teaching materials that everyone can share. Transparencies of sample pages of *MeSH* or a schematic of the search process may be used by a variety of classes.

Signs

Signs used for temporary promotional purposes are discussed in this section. (Information concerning use of signs as instructional aids is provided in Chapter 3.) There are a number of software programs written specifically for designing signs, banners, and flyers. Many have built-in graphics or clip art that can give a professional look to signs. If the library itself does not have access to such software, it may be available elsewhere in the institution, in other departments, or through commercial printing establishments. Another source of help for signs is *Marketing Treasures.* Three times a year this newsletter includes sheets of camera-ready library clip art. Collections of library clip art in print and electronic form are also available from the publisher of the newsletter. Some of these are geared specifically to health sciences libraries.

Signs can be posted in the library and in other public places such as lobbies, student unions, doctors' lounges, cafeterias, and meeting rooms. They can be suspended from the ceiling, mounted on easels, fastened to walls, or printed on balloons. Signs can also be displayed on computer screens.

Since these signs are for promotional purposes, it is important to remove them promptly when they are outdated. Otherwise, they lose their impact and cause confusion and clutter.

Information Sheets

Information sheets or flyers can accompany signs or be used alone. A sign can include a cardboard pocket for holding flyers. Sheets can be posted on bulletin boards, stuffed in mailboxes, left on library counters, or handed out by library staff. Some flyers will be location or time specific, such as "Using the Online Catalog" or a schedule of Fall classes.

The content of most information sheets should answer the questions of who, what, when, where, why, and how. When advertising a session, contact information and the name of the program can be printed on a section that can be torn off the bottom of the sheet, thus increasing the impact of the information sheet. The number of slips torn off at the time the sheets were removed would give a rough indication of interest in the topic.

Registration Forms

A registration requirement is helpful to the teacher, whether classes are offered free or for a fee. The users' names are less important than their departments and titles. Especially when teaching a complex subject like database searching, knowing the identity and disciplines of attendees can help in meeting their needs, choosing relevant examples, and teaching at the appropriate level. Registration information can also help when composing more homogeneous groups for small group work or hands-on sessions, if that is desired.

If a class is regularly oversubscribed, a waiting list may be useful. Those added to the list are informed that they will be contacted if space becomes available. Calling all registrants a day or two before the class will identify users that do not intend to come. These spaces can then be offered to those on the waiting list, thus ensuring that classes are fully subscribed and teaching resources used most efficiently. If the waiting list is small, one can suggest that those users turn up anyway and every effort will be made to accommodate them. Free classes always suffer from no-shows. It would be a shame if someone on the waiting list were denied entry when there was, in fact, space.

Latecomers can cause a problem if their places in class have been filled by those on the waiting list. Registration forms can carry a notation that, "Latecomers will not be admitted," or "Latecomers will be allowed to observe the class." Another option is for latecomers to be admitted but not participate in the hands-on portions. Every effort should be made to allow people to observe if they have come some distance or come in bad weather. Tactful and appropriate enforcement of such rules is important for the consideration of the other class participants and for precedent and consistency.

Classes involving hands-on work require registration if limited equipment or materials are being used. If the class is oversubscribed, the teacher can ask attendees who have come together to share equipment and materials. The teacher should follow this up by making sure anyone leaving without all the class materials receives a complete set as soon after the class as possible.

Classes may also be offered by appointment if attendance is expected to be small. This allows for greater flexibility in scheduling and better assurance that attendees will come.

Syllabi

Class attendees may not use what they have learned immediately [47]. They need comprehensive handouts and their own notes to refresh their memories at the time they try out what they have learned. Syllabi and handouts also say a great deal about the quality of teaching. They should be logical, comprehensive, and easy to read. A clear, consistent, and dignified style is important; correct spelling and grammar are compulsory.

Class syllabi and handouts should follow standard formats, with goals and learning objectives stated at the beginning and carefully spelled out. It is helpful to provide paper copies of transparencies in the handouts so that students can annotate them. A standard and attractive logo gives a professional look and helps unify the materials visually [48]. A color-coding system will help teachers and participants keep track of materials from different classes. Using different colors for the various handouts also helps participants find the items quickly and makes them visually attractive.

Meetings may be necessary to ensure that every teacher follows the syllabus and understands what additional content is included in the class. The syllabus should include the name of the library and appropriate addresses or telephone numbers for follow-up or additional information. Finally, if the syllabi and handouts carry a date and the initials of their authors, the need for updating and who is responsible will be obvious.

Cheat Sheets

There are occasions when the user wants brief, clear instructions that can be grasped quickly. Cheat sheets can help the user who has taken a class but needs a refresher, or the user who wants to do a simple search of the catalog or database but is short on time.

Cheat sheets are one-page sets of instructions that leave out rationale and more sophisticated techniques. The user who rarely comes to the library, knows nothing about computers, and wants to find a book in the online catalog or a few references in MEDLINE is a frequent user of these teaching aids. However, other types of users and participants of educational programs can benefit from these instructions as well.

Copies of cheat sheets can be left by workstations, mounted and laminated, or handed out by a busy reference librarian. Users can start helping themselves immediately while waiting for the librarian to assist them.

Evaluation Forms

It is useful to mention the management issues related to evaluations. Apart from the immediate value of feedback to the teacher, information from evaluation forms can make a useful database for future planning. Important information for planning includes

- Department of attendee.
- Status (e.g., faculty, student, nurse, staff).
- How the attendee heard about the program.
- Rating data on usefulness, organization, length.
- Yes or no response to "Would you recommend this course to colleagues?"
- Yes or no response to "Is this the first [name of library] education program you have attended?"
- Free-form responses for "What did you like most? and "What did you like least?"

Evaluation forms can be attached to the printed syllabus or handed out separately. For short-term evaluation, the forms should be brief and require few pen strokes to fill out. It is best to allow time in class for participants to complete the form, so there is a greater chance of collecting them. Users may be more honest if the form is anonymous.

Data, whether kept manually or electronically, can be used to publicize library activities, to compile librarians' dossiers, and to indicate trends in the library's user population. A well-designed database can provide statistics on the number of classes taught, number of students versus clinicians attending programs, the workload for a particular librarian, the total hours spent teaching, the percentage of total department work time spent teaching, and similar facts. The ACRL Bibliographic Instruction Section has published at least one list suggesting the types of statistics that may be useful to track [49].

Public sector and nonprofit organizations typically measure productivity using resources put into programs, rather than the traditional products described by the private sector. An example in education would be to report the amount of money being spent on a program, the number of specific classes or workshops offered, or the number of individuals participating. If librarians were to find more meaningful measures to describe educational services, it would profit them in terms of obtaining and allocating resources. This would require more complex and long-term follow-up of programs to determine results, but would provide compelling data to use in negotiating financial support for the library. Library users would have meaningful information about the value they could expect from the library, which would enhance their perception of the importance of the library to their professional efforts.

A database management program can be used for compiling these types of information. The library may have an integrated information management system that can link these data to other statistics such as registrations, user profiles, and overall reference workload. *Library Technology Reports* is a good source of reviews and comparisons of information management systems in the library context. Because the use of microcomputers and database management software is relatively widespread in health sciences libraries, this discussion centers on the use of that technology for data control.

If the database includes evaluation data as well as the course title, time of day, and teacher's initials, it is possible to ascertain whether a particular teacher is consistently rated as "clear" or "talks too fast," whether nurses rate a class higher than do students, and whether a particular time slot is popular. Summaries of comments from evaluation forms can also be a useful tool for convincing administrators of the value of the library's instructional programs.

Other practical considerations for data collection include attaching a cover sheet to each class' batch of forms, because students sometimes fill out the name of the class and the date incorrectly. The teacher, the instruction coordinator, or the department head may want to scan the forms before the information is put into the database. For the database to be statistically useful, the information should be as complete as possible. Entry procedures must be easy for clerical assistants to use and information should be entered on a regular basis so that the data reports are as current as possible. (For a more complete discussion of evaluation, refer to Chapter 5.)

Office Statistics

Evaluation and registration forms can be used to compile statistics on no-shows, money collected, numbers of handouts produced and distributed, and rooms and equipment used. A spreadsheet may be more appropriate for this purpose, especially for the financial data. The library's or the institution's administrative office may be interested in statistics rather than verbal comments. In an academic library, statistics may be collected for reporting to a national body such as the American Association of Health Sciences Library Directors (AAHSLD).

As with the comments from the evaluation forms, statistics can be used to demonstrate the usefulness and extent of the library's programs. They are also an advertising tool. A letter, for example, can be sent to new faculty pointing out that ten faculty members sent 200 students to the library last year to learn how to do research for their term papers. The new head of the hospital pharmacy can be invited to a demonstration of *International Pharmaceutical Abstracts* on CD-ROM because his predecessor had sent staff to the library regularly for the past five years to learn about new sources of pharmaceutical information.

Teaching Space

To a limited extent, physical facilities will determine how instruction will be carried out. However, a real effort should be made not to allow the library facilities to limit options. Educational services staff should prepare an instructional program that they think would best meet the instructional goals and objectives. Once that is done, they should seek out facilities, in the library or elsewhere, that best suit the planned instruction. Only when that has been done should changes be made to match the instructional design to the room space available [50].

In a library with a large user population and a classroom or lecture hall, the teaching style is more formal and addresses wider audiences. With a microcomputer classroom these lectures can be more personalized with the addition of hands-on computer practice sessions. If classroom space is not available, one-on-one instruction can be offered, perhaps on an appointment basis to accommodate everyone's busy schedule. The advantage of this kind of teaching is that it allows the librarian to create closer working relationships with users and to tailor instruction to their personal needs.

Teaching Materials

Hands-on practice is almost always desirable for any instruction in library use or information management. Superseded monthly/bimonthly copies of tools such as *Index Medicus* or *Science Citation Index* can be saved for class use. Larger libraries, not necessarily in the field of biomedicine, may subscribe to tools such as *Index Medicus* and be willing to donate their superseded copies. Vendors may be contacted for outdated print copies of indexing and abstracting tools. Some vendors, such as CINAHL Information Systems, produce teaching materials that libraries are welcome to use in educational programs; pages have already been made into transparencies or slides for classroom use. If the class involves a piece of software or a database, vendors may have related teaching materials available. If these are audiovisuals or instructional disks, they may be loaned to users if the librarian does not have the equipment to show it in the library.

Demo Codes and Disks

Online vendors are usually happy to provide demonstration codes for teaching and, as discussed above, often have free instructional materials to accompany them. The librarian who uses the software in class is indirectly promoting the product. Many software packages also have demo versions. To request these, it is worth sending a letter to software producers describing the class being taught, estimating the potential size of the audience, explaining that the software program will be demonstrated, and noting that attendees are potential purchasers. While the librarian may point out the good and bad points of various packages, it is difficult not to answer users' frequent insistence that the librarian recommend one package over another. (For a discussion of ethics, which should underlie these decisions, see Chapter 1.) The time and effort required to compare and evaluate the various packages is valuable to users and the librarian should not hesitate to make suggestions—provided, of course, that the librarian has investigated the subject thoroughly [51]. (For information on an electronic discussion list about personal bibliographic database management software, see Appendix C.) Further software issues are discussed in this chapter in the section on Microcomputer Centers and Learning Labs.

Scheduling

The library should contact the necessary offices in the academic schools or hospital units to obtain all schedules of classes, clinic hours, times for site visits and grand rounds, and any other information that will help determine when potential class attendees have free time. Offering the same class on different days and at different times gives attendees a choice. Lunch time is popular for brief demonstrations or tours, especially if food and drinks are allowed or provided. Friday afternoon programs are usually poorly attended because most people are anxious to start the weekend. Other scheduling considerations include avoiding the period right after lunch for classes in closed rooms in which the lights will be dim, for obvious reasons. It is more successful to schedule library programs at the end of class or clinic, rather than leave more than fifteen minutes between them. Students who finish a class at three, for example, will not want to wait until four to begin a library class.

Curriculum-related classes may be easier to control in this respect. Faculty can be asked to ensure that students adhere to a schedule, if more than one group of students is coming. Librarians can insist on a maximum size for each group sent to the library. It is frustrating to librarians and students alike if thirty turn up for a session arranged for twenty, the room is overcrowded, and not all the students have access to a computer or handouts.

Another scheduling method is to offer first-come-first-served classes at regular times and at regular locations, for example, in the online catalog area. If a public-address system is available, classes can be announced ten minutes before they start to increase attendance.

Innovative scheduling can include evening, weekend, and breakfast meetings, as well as tying instructional programs to other occasions such as a hospital open house or campus alumni day.

Economics and Fees

Direct costs of instructional programs may include room and equipment rental, hardware or software purchases, fees paid to outside instructors, staff time spent on preparation, teaching, and follow-up, online, printing, and telephone charges, refreshment costs, and reproduction of handouts. Indirect costs include building overhead, net increases or decreases in use of services as a result of instruction, and unbillable professional and support staff time. This last category might include expenses for staff development or benefits programs.

Economic factors related to instruction sometimes need investigation. A particular instructional program may appear to be too expensive, but analysis may reveal that, while front-end costs are high, they amortize quickly. When large dollar amounts are involved, librarians can outline scenarios that detail the costs and benefits of the alternatives. This is known as a risk assessment.

A potential benefit of investing in instructional services is to free up resources. An example using technology would be creating an expert system to provide library users with directional information, freeing staff from conducting tours or answering these questions at an information desk.

There is not a simple relationship between the cost of technology and time saved, nor is there an easy way to calculate the impact of technology on productivity [52]. There is fear, on occasion, that technology will replace people. That has not proved to be the case in the service sector [53]. The thoughtful application of technology provides an opportunity to increase services, either through reassigning people to other service areas or by creating new services. (For a description of recent and emerging technologies to consider, see Chapter 5.)

Next to the cost of technology, staff time is the other significant expense of providing educational services. Quantifying the costs of instruction has received little attention in the library literature, but King provides one analysis [54]. In the example he provides, "...the librarian's time accounts for almost two-thirds of the total cost of the instruction program" [55]. A rough way of figuring the amount of staff time required for a program is to estimate that for every hour of instruction, three to five hours of preparation and follow-up are needed. This ratio decreases the more times an instructor teaches the same class.

The costs of staff time must also be examined from a broader level. Administratively, decisions must be made that balance the information and document delivery roles of library staff with their educational roles. The degree of commitment to education will have a significant effect on what kind and what amount of fiscal and personnel resources are devoted to this effort [56].

There are three basic cost-recovery options for user education programs: offer free instruction and absorb all costs for materials and overhead; charge a materials fee that covers actual costs; or charge a larger fee and recoup some overhead costs as well as materials costs. The option chosen may be dictated by overall institutional policies.

Fees can vary according to user group. Individuals from outside the institution, for example, may be charged a fee for classes that are otherwise free. Tours, orientations, curriculum-related classes, and instruction related directly to using the library are usually offered free. Computer literacy, reprint file management, and other subjects less directly related to the library are more suitable candidates for fees because they typically involve special equipment, materials, or space.

Other fee income can be generated by educational programs. Libraries with education facilities may charge a rental fee for use of the rooms by nonlibrary staff. Syllabi can be sold both locally to users, whether attending classes or not, and nationally to other librarians or users. Consulting fees may be charged for extensive personal instruction that is beyond the scope of the library's regular programs.

Whether charging for consulting or not, the library will have to decide whether the considerable help being requested falls within existing service guidelines and can be offered during working hours. The library may decide that this is not within the bounds of current staff time and allow librarians to make their own private arrangements for consulting, provided there is no conflict of interest. Administrators must make a policy decision for cases in which library overhead costs would be incurred.

All fees should be stated in round figures that are easy to collect as cash. They should not be so small that checks or requisitions, or the effort to collect them, would be wasteful. Charging any kind of fee is believed to decrease the number of no-shows. Charging a fee will also put a psychological value on the class in the mind of the participant. Fees may also have a negative impact, discouraging students or others with limited income. If members of these groups are potential participants, their needs should be considered in choosing a fee structure. A fee assistance program or contacting an appropriate group to underwrite a program are options for low-income users.

Fee collection methods vary according to institutional policy. Purchase orders, departmental requisitions, or other internal payment methods may be the most expeditious. Some libraries may be unable to handle cash; many cannot accept credit cards. If all class participants are from the institution, not requiring identification when writing checks is a courtesy. Receipts should be made available to those who need them for reimbursement or tax purposes. Whatever methods are made available, payment instructions should be clearly listed on all flyers, schedules, and class announcements.

Any fees collected may be liable to sales or other taxes. This varies from state to state and from one institution to another. If the library has not sold printed materials or charged fees for classes before, fiscal officers from the institution should be consulted.

For more information on sources of financial support, budgeting, and cost-benefit analysis for educational services, see Zachert [57].

Microcomputer Centers and Learning Labs

What follows here is a discussion of the relationship of microcomputer centers and learning labs to educational services for users. For a comprehensive treatment of administration of these resources, see Hannigan and Brown's *Managing Public Access Microcomputers in Health Sciences Libraries* [58].

Role and Responsibility

Library use today requires basic computer literacy. Thus, it is essential to incorporate computers and related technology into library educational programs and to use teaching facilities which provide opportunities for hands-on instruction. Users will be less resistant to library automation if they are already comfortable with computers.

Just as libraries have traditionally been involved in self-education and literacy, they have a responsibility to teach users the skills they need to find the same information electronically that they had previously found in print sources. (For information on setting up a typical end-user training program, see Volume 1 of this series: *Reference and Information Services in Health Sciences Libraries.)*

Librarians hope that users of noncomputerized library resources can read and understand English; alphabetize; understand the difference between an author, a title, and a subject; grasp the concept of a thesaurus; understand special types of indexes such as KWIC/KWOC and citation indexing; know the difference between the primary literature and indexing services; and work with call numbers and classification systems. If users lack any of these skills, the library's role is to teach them. Indeed, some librarians may feel responsible for ensuring that users have these skills [59-61].

No matter how user-friendly the online catalog and its keyboard layout, using menus and locating keys such as *Enter* and *PrtSc* can be a mystery to some. Literature searching also requires considerable computer skills. Using Boolean operators, understanding the basics of database structure, and working with the mechanics of printing and downloading—are all easier with some understanding of operating systems or command languages. If the journal indexes are on CD-ROM but users have never used function keys or a mouse, the necessary computer skills are a prerequisite. For off-site users struggling with their own hardware and software, basic computer training is a must.

Some libraries have responded to users' needs for computer literacy training by offering classes in word processing, database management, desktop publishing, local area network (LAN) management, and electronic mail. This response has been particularly true in settings where no one else is able or willing to fill this void. Academic medical centers may be geographically separate from the rest of the university. The physicians and students who use a hospital library may be far removed from any other facility.

Other libraries have been able to refer users to locally available computer literacy classes. Still others have fashioned cooperative programs with computing centers elsewhere in the institution, sharing the costs of design, printing, teaching, and so forth [62-63].

Both learning and teaching new technology is time-consuming. Organizing classes and advertising them to users takes time, in addition to the hours spent teaching. Time is needed for maintenance of hardware, loading upgrades of software, and troubleshooting the inevitable "bugs" and problems that occur with computerized systems. These issues will be addressed in this section as they relate to educational programs.

Promoting Computer Literacy Programs

As with other types of instruction, computer literacy programs need to be targeted to specific audiences. Employing the five steps of marketing will ensure that this is accomplished.

The following examples illustrate the attitudes of different levels of users and suggest techniques to use when promoting computer literacy to each of them.

Example: Professionals may have closet resistance to becoming computer literate for various reasons. They may feel there is too much to learn or be intimidated in front of a keyboard. Administrators and supervisors may see word processing as an extension of typing and regard library work as secretarial. Some users may never have learned, or long since forgotten, how to type. Others may secretly wish to know what their colleagues are talking about but think the learning curve is too steep and do not know where to begin. These individuals have to be convinced that becoming familiar with a keyboard is a suitably professional thing to do.

An introduction to the mysteries of computing should take place in a nonthreatening setting. One way to persuade health professionals that they can feel comfortable in front of a monitor and keyboard is to enlist colleagues in the health professions who are already at ease with this activity. Another way is to show the uninitiated a few articles that discuss health professionals searching for themselves [64-68]. Literature from vendors who target clinicians can be used. Wary physicians and faculty can be invited for special training with only their peers present. Librarians may suggest going to clinics or offices for a one-on-one first session, then invite them to gather a group of colleagues together for further training. Carefully worded invitations can attract those without prior experience with computers.

Example: Every year, more incoming students, interns, and residents have already had computer training in school or college. If not, they too must be persuaded that they need it. Either way, when they finish training, they will be better prepared for their future if they are comfortable with computers.

Students can be reached in a variety of ways:

- *Faculty support.* The librarian has a captive audience if class assignments include completing computer-assisted lessons or providing proof that the students have done their own computer literature search.
- *Impressive papers.* Students can be lured by promises of better term papers and easy access to knowledge about the latest case studies, guaranteed to impress their professors.
- *Less work.* The benefits of beautifully word-processed papers or the attractiveness of scanning the latest journals without actually turning any pages can be emphasized.

The librarian can reach interns and residents by focusing on patient care applications. Offering to do free searches can gain their attention, followed by instruction on how to use a microcomputer to search the library's CD-ROM network or the locally mounted database. Researching a surgical procedure or dosage regimen without leaving the clinic has obvious promotional value.

The following scenario points out many of the opportunities found in health sciences libraries for introducing users to computerized information management.

SCENARIO: Dr. X has learned to search MEDLINE on CD-ROM in the library. She has also learned how to download retrieval into a file. Now, she wants to know how to organize the references. The librarian suggests various software programs. Dr. X would also like paper copies of some of the articles. The librarian explains how Dr. X can keep track of both hard copies and references in the software program. The doctor's MEDLINE search was related to a clinical trial in which she is involved. She is helping prepare the manuscript. The librarian shows her how to incorporate references from her downloaded database into the manuscript.

Colleagues whom Dr. X met at a recent conference have told her that the cryptic codes on their business cards are e-mail. She asks the librarian what this means and how she can have access to it. The library offers a class on using electronic mail. Dr. X is leaving the city and moving to a rural area. The librarian tells her how she can continue to search MEDLINE and obtain copies of articles through the GRATEFUL MED software's automated document delivery option, LOANSOME DOC. Before she leaves the area,

Dr. X attends a library class intended for those who are graduating or leaving and who will no longer have the library's searching facilities available. The class explains how modems and telecommunications software work and gives practical advice for those who will be setting up such systems by themselves.

Each step taken by this imaginary clinician is an educational opportunity. Examples from this scenario can be incorporated into promotional materials and presentations for specific programs.

Microcomputer Classrooms

The hospital librarian without support staff cannot take time to go to each user's office with a computer and software to demonstrate its use. The large library on a sprawling campus may not have staff to provide one-on-one instruction at remote sites, except in exceptional cases. One solution in these situations is a microcomputer center. It can be as modest as a single workstation with a modem or network connection. The librarian can hold demonstrations and invite attendees to come back individually for hands-on practice. The following is a series of increasingly sophisticated arrangements for microcomputer centers.

- A room (or section of a room) with tables and chairs, or desks, a chalkboard (or other board with markers), and a microcomputer.
- A room (or section of a room) with a microcomputer, modem or network connection, telephone line, and a monitor large enough to be seen by a small number of attendees.
- A means of projecting from the instructor's microcomputer to a large screen.
- Provision of microcomputers for all class attendees for hands-on training.
- Networking all the workstations together so that software may be shared, usage statistics kept, and students' screens can be examined on the instructor's screen.

Hardware and Equipment Considerations

The first consideration when discussing hardware is money for continual upgrading and improvement. If a library received a grant five years ago to set up a microcomputer learning lab with personal computers (PCs), floppy disk drives, monochrome monitors, and 1200-baud modems, it will be severely handicapped today. New versions of software require larger capacity memory, monitors with graphics capabilities, and upgraded printers. In the teaching environment, it is particularly important that students learn with and about the latest technology. It may be possible for a library to isolate itself and continue to use older equipment, but in the world of networking, this is impractical. User education must look beyond the immediate goal of teaching skills useful in-house to the greater goal of lifelong learning. To teach users how to take advantage of the latest technology, the library must have a budget for upgrading hardware and software.

Institutional volume discounts, site licenses, and discounts on upgrades should all be investigated when purchasing software. The library has some leverage with vendors because it will be teaching potential purchasers. Agreements and contracts should be read carefully. An institutional volume discount may require that the library persuade a certain number of users to purchase the program within a given time period. Site licenses may restrict usage to affiliated members of the institution; a library may have to require that a library card and identification be produced before anyone is given access to a program or database.

Networking can help the small hospital library expand its resources. Even if the library has only one modest workstation, it can be connected to an institutional network so that users can access modem pools, electronic mail connections, and computer-assisted instructional programs that would not be available on the stand-alone workstation. The librarian in this situation should feel comfortable dealing with the institution's computer departments and be fully conversant with the programs that are available.

Medical centers may have satellite broadcast facilities that provide an electronic classroom situation. Remote projection from other sites where classes are being held enables participants to watch the instructor, call in with their questions, and sometimes use an electronic blackboard to write comments and requests. The institution receiving the programs has a satellite dish and classrooms or conference rooms for displaying the programs. The Hospital Satellite Network provides services of this kind. The Veterans' Administration has a program for its hospitals. Other sources are the American Hospital Association and commercial interests such as pharmaceutical companies. Many of the programs are for continuing medical education, nurses' training, and other hospital staff training. The National Library of Medicine also transmits pertinent programs on library services.

The larger academic library faces different issues. Classroom equipment is a big investment but offers valuable teaching opportunities. A classroom allows students to take notes, to ask questions, and to help one another. To make sessions interesting, the teacher may lecture for awhile and then allow time for discussion and personal experimentation and practice. Isolated from other library users in a separate room, students can concentrate on the subject at hand. Distraction for other library users is eliminated. Education programs are greatly enhanced by provision of large-screen projectors and sufficient workstations for all participants to have simultaneous hands-on training, monitored by the teacher or an assistant. Some network arrangements allow the teacher to view individual students' screens on the teacher's own monitor or broadcast messages or help screens to the class as a whole.

Provision of printing for class attendees can be a major expense. Unless print commands are a vital part of the instruction, it may not be necessary to provide printing during class. This decision must be weighed against the very positive reaction attendees have when they can take personally interesting results home with them. An alternative to printing is downloading to a disk that users purchase or bring with them. Attendees may then take the disk back to the office for printing.

Users can be trained to be conservative in their printing, either through mechanical restraints or written or verbal instruction. Some CD-ROM producers, for example, allow installers to limit the number of references printed at one time. Another solution is to have a large shared printer to which users can direct their retrieval. Users pay by the page for their printouts when they request them at the service desk. Whether printing is allowed at all, how much, on what kind of printer, and for what cost must be determined by the library and the details must be incorporated into education programs so that users know exactly what is available.

For user education, the classroom workstations need access to the systems being taught, whether through networks or dial-up telecommunications. Sufficient ports must be available for simultaneous access for the maximum number of participants planned. The classroom should be tested by booting up all the stations simultaneously and having every station send an identical command (search retrieval or printing, for example) at the same moment, to ensure that the system can cope. Significant loss of operating speed or even jamming of the system should be identified before students try it out!

Maintenance and troubleshooting can be time-consuming and require skills most librarians have not gained as part of their regular training. Presentations at professional meetings, electronic discussion lists, and the literature of librarianship and microcomputing abound with advice on how to establish and maintain support for these essential functions. Classroom equipment must be monitored constantly to be kept in full working order. Problems with drives, keyboards, and monitors should be repaired or reported immediately and maintenance of classroom equipment should be a priority. Whoever maintains the workstations must also ensure that the hard disks or diskettes are checked regularly for files created during class that may fill the disks or cause other problems. If students practice downloading, for example, or manipulate a sample file loaded on a diskette, the drives and disks must be restored to their original state after class. Even if boot disks are protected, students may remove the tabs and inadvertently format the boot diskette or erase necessary program files. Teachers should always have extra copies of diskettes available and be prepared to deal with system crashes and error messages caused by students.

Various backup arrangements should be in place. For example, if using Ethernet connections, some stations may be equipped with modems for when the Ethernet is down. Instructors may want to have overhead transparencies and printed indexes handy for when electronic systems fail. If the class involves the use of passwords, keep extras on hand for emergencies such as when students reboot the station in the middle of a search and make the password temporarily unavailable.

Uniformity and standardization are important. All the keyboards should be identical in layout, and the stations should have the same power and speed. The teacher's own station should be able to project its image on a large screen or wall. When learning complicated commands, students can see what the teacher is doing and repeat the steps. It is important that the classroom workstations operate just as students' own computers will operate and reflect what they will experience when they take their newly learned skills back to the home, clinic or office. If the training includes installing software or booting up the station, any differences between the classroom stations and other types the user may encounter should be explained.

A classroom with microcomputers and display equipment enables students to experience the most highly rated component of computer classes—hands-on practice. The best way to overcome the fear of computers and to understand what happens when the keys are tapped is to sit in front of a keyboard with a teacher guiding the action and actually *do it!* Students can see what the teacher is typing on the screen, then copy the command themselves. If an assistant teacher is watching what students type and helping when they go astray, the pace of instruction will be lively.

Computer Class Participants

As with other instruction, homogenous groups are easier to teach. This is particularly important with computers. Those who cannot type or understand English well, or who are intimidated by computers, can impede the progress of others. The particular skills needed depend on the type of microcomputers being used. For example, if the instruction will be using DOS-based machines, participants need to be familiar with the keyboard, particularly the function keys, Ctrl, Alt, and the numerical pad. In a Macintosh or Windows environment, participants must be comfortable with using a mouse and understand the concepts of buttons and scroll-bars.

The library could offer a brief preliminary class with a title such as, "Basics of Microcomputing" or "Introduction to the Macintosh." If there is a computer department nearby that offers similar courses, the library can schedule and advertise its own classes so that participants learn the basics prior to taking the library's courses. It is important that the interval be brief between the basic course and more advanced classes so that what is learned is put to immediate use.

Support Staff

Even librarians with a high level of computer expertise are unlikely to be able to spend a large part of their working days with screwdrivers and cables in their pockets, troubleshooting and maintaining large numbers of workstations, local area networks, CD-ROM towers, and dumb terminals. The library that has had microcomputers for many years and has gradually added to their numbers and sophistication will probably have outgrown its ability to provide in-house expertise with existing staff and have discovered the need for additional help. Depending on library size and resources, employees may be hired for this purpose or consultants may be brought in from other departments in the institution.

There are some major advantages to having full-time experts as library employees. They are there when needed for maintenance and troubleshooting; they can teach users and library staff; they can advise on the purchase of upgrades and new hardware and software; and they enhance the image of the library as a place where all aspects of information management are addressed.

However, the library needs to be prepared for the situation in which the experts' skills and advice become so popular that their responsibilities have to be restricted. For example, the library's role may be to help users install communications software but not to help them connect to online shopping malls. The library may teach users to download MEDLINE retrieval and import it into a database management program but not to help with medical records or personal finances. The library may also have to decide that its experts only help users who come into the library or call by telephone rather than sending the experts out to remote sites to help with assorted word processing problems. Ideally, library administrators would seek additional support to respond to requests that are related to information management.

Summary

This chapter has attempted to describe how health sciences libraries currently administer educational programs, to make recommendations based on the experiences of a wide variety of librarians, and to emphasize that almost any library can offer such programs for the benefit of its users.

Proponents of universally available user-friendly information systems state that computer literacy training would not be necessary if systems were better designed [69-71]. This utopia is not yet upon us and, until it is, libraries must provide the education that health professionals need to take advantage of all the forms of information that are available.

Even a brief review of articles written in such publications as the *Bulletin of the Medical Library Association* or *Medical Reference Services Quarterly,* of papers presented at local and national meetings of health sciences librarians, or of continuing education syllabi at these meetings, reveals that user education is a standard part of the operation of many libraries. Training of some kind in the use of computers is usually a part of this education. This discussion has assumed, therefore, that librarians should and do teach users to help themselves to find information in all its available formats. The investments in time, training, equipment, materials, and effort will be rewarded by rapport with users, a sense of personal and professional achievement, and, most of all, the knowledge that these health professionals will be better equipped to find the information they need to improve health care.

References

1. Bunyan LE, Lutz EM. Marketing the hospital library to nurses. Bull Med Libr Assoc 1991 Apr;79(2):223-5.

2. Schwartz DG. Bibliographic instruction: a public relations perspective. Med Ref Serv Q 1984 Summer;3(2):43-9.

3. Gilbert CM. Challenges in health care information transfer: the role of hospital libraries. Bull Med Libr Assoc 1991 Oct;79(4):406.

4. Baker B, Sandore B, Larson ME, Hensley R. Educational roles for academic libraries. Coll Res Libr News 1989 Dec;50(11):987.

5. Zachert MJ, Williams RV. Marketing measures for information services. Spec Libr 1986 Spring;77(2):61-70.

6. Strauss D. Marketing fundamentals for librarians. NC Libr 1988 Fall;46(3):132-5.

7. Ibid., 134.

8. Kotler P. Principles of marketing. 3d ed. Englewood Cliffs, NJ: Prentice-Hall, 1986:757.

9. McGinn HF. Libraries and marketing: new words—old worlds. NC Libr 1988 Fall;46(3):126-31.

10. Ciliberti AC, Casserly MF, Hegg JL, Mitchell ES. Material availability: a study of academic library performance. Coll Res Libr 1987 Nov;48(6):513-27.

11. Kolner SJ, Welch EC. The book availability study as an objective measure of performance in a health sciences library. Bull Med Libr Assoc 1985 Apr;73(2):121-31.

12. Gothberg HM. The library survey: a research methodology rediscovered. Coll Res Libr 1990 Nov;51(6):553-9.

13. Schlichter DJ, Pemberton JM. The emperor's new clothes? Problems of the user survey as a planning tool in academic libraries. Coll Res Libr 1992 May;53(3):257-65.

14. Sirkin AF. Marketing planning for maximum effectiveness. Spec Libr 1991 Winter;82(1):1-6.

15. Katz WA. Introduction to reference work. Volume II: reference services and reference processes. 5th ed. New York: McGraw-Hill, 1987:41-3.

16. Bregman A, Mento B. Reference roving at Boston College. Coll Res Libr News 1992 Nov;53(10):634-7.

17. Pfeiffer S, Algermissen V. A unique heavy users forum: a program to involve a library's most frequent users. Med Ref Serv Q 1992 Fall;11(3):17-27.

18. Nelson JL. An analysis of transaction logs to evaluate the educational needs of end users. Med Ref Serv Q 1992 Winter;11(4):11-21.

19. Patterson TH. Library skills workshops for support personnel. RQ 1980 Summer;19(4):351-3.

20. Edwards A. Organizational process for a secretarial and research assistants' workshop. Med Ref Serv Q 1989 Spring;8(1):72.

21. Zachert, op. cit., 63.

22. Cooper ER. Marketing the hospital library to physicians: one approach. Bull Med Libr Assoc 1991 Jan;79(1):86-7.

23. Zachert, op. cit., 66-9.

24. Cargill JS. Cooperative cohabitation: libraries and computer learning centers. Libr Soft Rev 1987 Nov/Dec;6(6):344-8.

25. Allegri F. Administrative structures for education programs. Med Ref Serv Q 1991 Summer;10(2):95-101.

26. Hubbard A, Wilson B. An integrated information management education program...defining a new role for librarians in helping end-users. Online 1986 Mar;10(2):16-8.

27. Self PC. User education in academic health sciences libraries: results of a survey. Med Ref Serv Q 1990 Winter;9(4):101-8.

28. Feng CCH, Weise FO. Part III. Implementation of integrated information services: library/computer center partnership. J Am Soc Info Sci 1988 Mar;39(2):129.

29. Wood EH. Symposium on staffing issues and public-access computer systems. Public Access Comput Syst Rev 1990;1(2):15-49.

30. Hubbard, op. cit., 16-7.

31. Broadwell MM. Ten myths about instructor training. Training 1990 May;27(5):81-83.

32. Medical Library Association. Platform for change: the educational policy statement of the Medical Library Association. Chicago: Medical Library Association, [1991]:[16].

33. Ibid., [11-7].

34. Bibliographic Instruction Section. American Library Association. Appendix C: proficiencies and competencies needed. In: Roberts AF, Blandy SG. Library instruction for librarians. 2d ed. rev. Englewood, CO: Libraries Unlimited, 1989:216-20.

35. Miller MI, Bratton BD. Instructional design: increasing the effectiveness of bibliographic instruction. Coll Res Libr 1988 Nov;49(6):545-9.

36. Warnken PN, Young VL. Application of training principles and techniques for successful library instruction. Ref Serv Rev 1991 Winter;19(4):91-6.

37. Bowden VM, Bierschenk NF, Olivier ER. Medical library employer expectations. J Libr Admin 1989;11(3/4):138-40.

38. Breivik PS. Information literacy: revolution in the library. New York: American Council on Education, Macmillan, 1989.

39. Presidential Committee on Information Literacy. American Library Association. Final Report. Chicago: American Library Association, 1989.

40. Roper FW, Mayfield MK, eds. Symposium: Platform for change: medical library education in the information age. Bull Med Libr Assoc 1993 Oct;81(4):393-432.

41. Tiefel V. Developing a teaching effectiveness program for librarians: the Ohio State University experience. Med Ref Serv Q 1988;7(4):78-86.

42. Planning and administering bibliographic instruction programs. CE 606. Chicago: Medical Library Association. 1993.

43. Ericksen SC. The essence of good teaching. San Francisco: Jossey Bass, 1984:135-7.

44. Ibid., 138-40.

45. Broadwell, op. cit., 82.

46. Stigleman S. Organizing information management education materials. Med Ref Serv Q 1991 Fall;10(3):61-6.

47. Eisenstaedt RF, Barry WE, Glanz K. Problem-based learning: cognitive retention and cohort traits of randomly selected participants and decliners. Acad Med 1990 Sept;65(9)Suppl:S11-2.

48. Olson CA. Test your library's marketing IQ. Med Ref Serv Q 1993 Fall;12(3):75-83.

49. Research Committee. Bibliographic Instruction Section. Association of College and Research Libraries. American Library Association. BI statistics tips. Coll Res Libr News 1984 Feb;45(2):86-7.

50. Hannigan GG, Brown JF. User services. In: Hannigan GG, Brown JF. Managing public access microcomputers in health sciences libraries. Chicago: Medical Library Association, 1990:115-7.

51. Stigleman S. Text management software. Public Access Comput Syst Rev 1990;1(1):5-22.

52. Riggs DE. Productivity increases in public services: are expert systems the answer? J Libr Admin 1988;9(4):97-8.

53. Senker J, Senker P. Gaining competitive advantage from information technology. J Gen Manage 1992 Spring;17(3):31-45.

54. King DN. Creating educational programs in libraries. Med Ref Serv Q 1988;7(1):67-76.

55. Ibid., 69.

56. Ibid., 75-6.

57. Zachert MJK. Educational services in special libraries: planning and administration. Chicago: Medical Library Association, 1990:100-106, 152-3, 164-5.

58. Hannigan GG, Brown JF. Managing public access microcomputers in health sciences libraries. Chicago: Medical Library Association, 1990.

59. Reichel M. Library literacy: refocusing and library instruction. RQ 1991 Summer;30(4):500-1.

60. Allegri F. Editorial comment: what is "information literacy"? Med Ref Serv Q 1987 Spring;6(1):95-7.

61. Wilson LA. Instruction as a reference service. In: Bopp RE, Smith LC, eds. Reference and information services: an introduction. Englewood, CO: Libraries Unlimited, 1991:120. (Library Science Text Series.)

62. Feng, op. cit., 126-30.

63. Shedlock J. Who's responsible for teaching information management? Med Ref Serv Q 1986 Summer;5(2):80.

64. Simpson RL. Brainpower at your fingertips: the National Library of Medicine. Nurs Manage 1991 Dec;22(12):14,16.

65. Cushing M, Jr. SilverPlatter literature searches. MD Comput 1992 May/Jun;9(3):178-80.

66. Lindberg DAB et al. Use of MEDLINE by physicians for clinical problem solving. JAMA 1993 Jun 23/30;269(24):3124-9.

67. Kelly JA, Hillson SD. Searching for answers: using computers to find the literature you need for patient care. Minn Med 1992 Oct;75(10):39-41.

68. Haynes RB et al. How to keep up with the medical literature: v. access by personal computer to the medical literature. Ann Int Med 1986 Nov;105(5):810-24.

69. Ensor P. On the conference circuit: Online/CD-Rom 1991. Technicalities 1991 Nov;11(11):6.

70. Nelson TH. The once and future literature. J Inf Sci 1990;16(6):339-43.

71. Gorman M. Send for a child of four! or creating the BI-less academic library. Libr Trends 1991 Winter;39(3):354-62.

5

Evaluation and Future Trends

Karla Hahn, Nadia J. Martin, and
Diane G. Schwartz

Stagnation is a danger faced by any program, and educational services are not immune. Often, educational programs are designed with a great deal of enthusiasm and may meet with considerable success. Two key ingredients will ensure that a successful instructional program will be sustained: ongoing managed evaluation and close monitoring of future trends in instructional methods and technology. These two provide instructors with the information needed to avoid boredom for themselves and irrelevancy for their trainees.

Evaluation aims to make the best possible match between users' needs and a program's resources. Yet, even with continuous, high quality evaluation, a class or an entire instructional program can become worthless if the instructor or program manager fails to respond to changes in resources and users' needs.

As instructors, librarians must also be alert to changes in information technology and medical librarianship. Monitoring trends in health care instruction, research, and practice is important as well. This awareness is necessary to determine the impact these changes will have on educational services and to make adjustments to instructional programs and methods.

Evaluation is often overlooked and undervalued. In a study of 122 public libraries in California, 94% of the respondents had not evaluated their services or programs within the last three years. Of those which had conducted evaluations, 78% had not yet initiated any of the suggested changes [1]. Given the common goal all libraries share of providing timely, high quality instruction, it is unfortunate that evaluation is overlooked as a means of obtaining the information needed to improve instructional services. Librarians frequently complain about how much there is to teach and how little time is available for instruction. Evaluation can help instructors make the most efficient and effective use of that limited time.

Goals and objectives form the basis for evaluation. (For information on writing goals and objectives, see Chapter 2.) The first part of this chapter will concentrate on the aims of evaluation, the types of evaluation, the steps involved, who should conduct evaluations, and the resources for designing data collection instruments.

As information services and users' needs change, effective instruction requires constant surveillance of the environment in which instruction occurs. This chapter's second section will describe trends in information technology, along with other changes affecting instructional services. The discussion will include pressures arising both from within and outside the health sciences library profession.

The Process of Evaluation

Evaluation is effective in determining the quality of services and measuring success in meeting predetermined objectives. The stumbling block for many librarians is that they do not know how, what, when, or whom to evaluate. A useful approach, outlined by the Bibliographic Instruction Section (BIS) of the American Library Association, is to divide evaluation into six steps:

1. Describe the purpose of the evaluation.
2. Describe the current program in terms of its goals and objectives.
3. Determine the evaluation criteria.
4. Develop the evaluation procedures and overall design of the study.
5. Develop instruments and collect data.
6. Analyze data and report results [2].

These steps are illustrated here in an example of an instructor evaluating a library orientation class for incoming house officers.

Example: The *purpose* of the evaluation could be to assess the timeliness and relevance of the information provided. The librarian wants to ensure a close match between the instructional presentation and the users' needs.

Completing the second step results in this stated *goal:* the program is to teach house officers the mechanics of using the library's online public access catalog (OPAC).

The next step is the determination of the *evaluation criteria.* Evaluation criteria are specific and measurable knowledge, skills, or abilities that can be gained from instructional programs or materials. In this case, the criteria could include knowledge of what is contained in the OPAC, the ability to perform a search using appropriate terminology and search strategies, and the ability to locate recent textbooks in a specified subject area.

The fourth step, the development of *evaluation procedures* and overall *study design,* is one of the most important in the evaluation process. Before this step can be completed successfully, the purpose or goals of the evaluation must be decided. If the study is not well designed, or an inappropriate evaluation method is used, the results may not be an accurate description of the effectiveness of the program or material. For the purposes of this example, the evaluation procedure used is a test to determine the house officers' knowledge of OPAC.

The fifth step in evaluation is *developing instruments and collecting data* from the study. Qualitative and quantitative data should be gathered. Quantitative data could be collected using a brief quiz at the end of class to measure the percentage of house officers who can successfully interpret a textbook record from the OPAC. Qualitative data could be collected with a brief survey asking the house officers if they felt they could immediately use the information presented in the instructional session.

The final step is to *analyze* and synthesize the data and *report and use* the results to improve the instructional program. In this example, the data might show that while many house officers could interpret a textbook record, they were unsure about selecting appropriate journal records and had difficulty in figuring out which volumes were owned by the library. Using this information, the class could then be revised to include a section on reading journal records and interpreting library holdings statements.

The Goals of Evaluation

All well-designed instructional programs have clearly defined goals and objectives. The evaluation process must have the same. Instructors undertake evaluation to accomplish one or more aims:

- To determine how the instruction affects knowledge, attitudes, or skills.
- To assess the skills and performance of the instructor.
- To convey the overall value of an instructional program or some part of it.

Thus, the first step in any effective evaluation plan is to determine the aims (i.e., the reasons) for designing and implementing an evaluation. As described above, these aims usually fall into three areas: learning domains, instructor performance, and program effectiveness.

Learning Domains

Often, the overall goal of educational programs is increased user self-sufficiency. As a result, a common goal of evaluation is to measure the learners' success in achieving *cognitive, affective,* and *psychomotor* objectives. (For more information on the different types of objectives, see Chapter 2.)

Cognitive skills deal with the recall of knowledge and the achievement of skills [3]. An example of a cognitive skill is a reader's ability to analyze critically an article purporting to describe a cure for cancer. Bloom's *Taxonomy of Educational Objectives* divides cognitive skills into six increasingly complex classes: knowledge, comprehension, application, analysis, synthesis, and evaluation [4]. Generally, higher-level cognitive skills, such as synthesis or analysis, are more difficult to evaluate than lower-order skills, such as knowledge.

As with goals for the acquisition of cognitive skills, instructors may also have goals to influence *affective* behaviors or attitudes. For instance, a librarian may want to reduce computer phobia in library users who believe that electronic databases are overrated as research tools. Conversely, the librarian may want to change the attitude of library users who have unrealistically high expectations about the type and quantity of material that can be retrieved by a computer search. A librarian may want both types of users to leave an instructional session with more realistic expectations. Quality instructional programs strive to alter attitudes as well as cognitive skills.

In comparison to intellectual and attitudinal abilities, *psychomotor* skills are easier to evaluate but are frequently overlooked. These are the skills used for physical and spatial tasks. For example, if people cannot confidently and successfully navigate computer keyboards, they will be increasingly frustrated with their inability to use effectively the library and its resources.

Instructor Performance

Another common goal when evaluating educational services is to monitor instructor performance. It is important to gather information on instructor performance to promote consistency and quality. This is particularly important if several different instructors present the same material.

The information gathered allows one to identify weaknesses in the instructor's preparation, presentation style, mastery of the subject matter, or ability to interact effectively with the class.

Program Effectiveness

Finally, overall program value can be the focus of evaluation. Educational services are costly. An effort needs to be made to determine the benefits that are achieved by following particular instructional strategies. Hernon and McClure have defined cost-benefit analysis as the method used to justify the expense of offering a service or program vis-a-vis the benefits that can be derived from it [5]. A cost-benefit focus to evaluation requires a long-term, comprehensive approach. To be comprehensive, a cost-benefit analysis should include overhead such as clerical and professional staff time required for instructional preparation and teaching. A comprehensive analysis also needs to include the cost of supplies such as paper, disks, slides, transparencies, and photocopying.

The goals of evaluation are not mutually exclusive, nor does a person need to choose only one to conduct an effective evaluation. Evaluation goals are selected to meet the needs of the library. However, once one or more goals have been identified, it is helpful to understand the three common types of evaluation and the role each type plays in the development of quality service.

Types of Evaluation

There are three common types of evaluation: formative, summative, and long-term. Each type of evaluation has different strengths and weaknesses for achieving certain evaluation goals.

Formative Evaluation

Formative evaluation focuses on program development [6]. Its goal is to help the librarian create effective educational materials and programs. Formative evaluation can identify problems with materials and strengthen educational goals and objectives. It is best activated at the beginning of the planning process, when a program or material is first being considered for use [7].

Analysis, design, evaluation, and revision are the four sequential steps in the formative evaluation process [8]. Initially, the instructor analyzes user needs or perceived needs. Should a class on how to use *Hospital Literature*

Index be required, or could the same objective be met with a point-of-use handout? Materials and classes are then designed which match predetermined objectives. The design takes into account such factors as time constraints, available staff and funds, knowledge level of users, and difficulty of the material. For example, users may need to attend a class on Medical Subject Headings (MeSH) structure before they can perform successful and relevant searches on MEDLINE.

Testing the teaching methodology with a small subset of the target population is an integral part of the formative evaluation process. This is frequently called a pilot test or pilot program. The pilot group should be asked to examine the clarity of the content, the pacing of the material, the amount of information presented, and the level of the presentation.

Incorporating suggested changes is just as important as gathering feedback. To complete the initial evaluation process, the class is revised to include the suggestions made by the pilot group. This process can be repeated as needed, with the final evaluation being done by the target audience.

The value of formative evaluation lies in its ability to reliably produce high-quality instruction tailored to fit the needs and background of the user group. Another advantage of this type of evaluation is that it promotes experimentation—the cost of failure is held to a minimum by the use of small pilot groups.

Summative Evaluation

Whereas, formative evaluation can be applied to the development process, summative evaluation is concerned with the overall effectiveness of a program or of specific instructional materials. For instance, can students successfully use *International Nursing Index* to find articles of value on their research topic? This type of evaluation is usually conducted at the end of an instructional program and uses a survey or questionnaire to collect data. Hernon and McClure note that summative evaluation, at its most basic level, determines the degree of program success or failure [9]. Most librarians are familiar with, and have used, summative evaluation to assess programs and materials.

While summative evaluation is sometimes easier and less time-consuming to conduct than formative or long-term evaluation, it is less valuable for improving instructional programs or materials. Summative evaluation is a snapshot of a program at a particular time. It can be helpful in deciding the following:

- Whether a program should be repeated.
- What a program's overall value is for resource allocation.
- Whether a program promotes positive public relations for the library.

Formative evaluation, on the other hand, has greater potential for improving the overall effectiveness of programs.

Long-term Evaluation

Long-term or ongoing evaluation fills the gap left by summative and formative evaluations. It is conducted regularly throughout the life of a program, and the data is collectively analyzed. This analysis provides a means of tracking the success or failure of a program over time, while providing a mechanism for quality control. As an example, if many of the staff teach end users to search MEDLINE, ongoing evaluation can ensure that all students receive the same degree of training. Another major benefit of long-term evaluation is its ability to inform librarians of users' changing needs. For example, it can record the level of computer literacy of incoming students so that instruction for these students can be adjusted accordingly.

Ongoing evaluation is a means of measuring the quality of instruction by providing feedback on whether class objectives are consistently met. Long-term evaluation is best suited for programs or instructional materials which are presented repeatedly, such as GRATEFUL MED instruction or handouts on how to use the online catalog. It usually takes the form of surveys, searching logs, or interviews. Like formative evaluation, long-term evaluation can be a time-consuming process, but it ensures that programs and materials evolve and adapt to changing user needs.

Formative, summative, and long-term evaluation each offer considerable benefits in return for the investment of time they require. Fortunately, they are not mutually exclusive. They can be used in tandem as tools for designing and fine-tuning instructional programs and materials.

What to Evaluate

Selecting which aspects of educational programs to target requires knowledge of an institution's goals for evaluation in addition to an understanding of the basic types of evaluation. The Continuing Education Committee of BIS has published a checklist of items to be evaluated when organizing and managing an instructional program. The list includes the following parameters: program content, products, process, instructors, attitude toward the library, efficiency or cost effectiveness, and overall quality [10]. Werking provides additional items for consideration: user performance, attitude toward librarians, position of instructional program within the library and the institution, and the priority assigned to instructional programs [11]. These two lists provide specific areas of concentration when trying to reach evaluation goals in the three areas of learning domains, instructor performance, and program effectiveness.

Many librarians choose an educational goal of increasing user self-sufficiency. When evaluating this goal, librarians tend to focus on user performance as it reflects cognitive learning. Unfortunately, it is often difficult to measure high-level cognitive performance, even though this is usually what most interests the instructor. Questions such as, "Are the students able to apply the class to their own information use problems?", can be difficult to answer. Various factors can influence performance, including the method of evaluation. In addition, those evaluation techniques which rely on self-reporting, such as point-of-use questionnaires, may only reach a small segment of the group being studied. More productive topics to study for user performance evaluation include the basic knowledge or skills users have before and after instruction, for example, typing skills or knowledge of MeSH descriptors. Questions on these topics can form a part of a formative evaluation program. For summative evaluation, questions can be asked that determine what factual information was learned during the instructional session.

As with high-level cognitive skills, affective skills or attitudes also pose challenges to evaluators. This is because attitudes can be influenced by unknown variables, such as previous library experience or level of computer literacy. Attitudes influence behavior. For example, a person who cannot type may be embarrassed to use a CD-ROM product. It can be difficult to measure the relationship between attitudes and behavior, as attitudes are implicit and learned [12].

Furthermore, it has been observed by behavioral psychologists that self-reported behavior differs from objectively observed behavior [13]. Analysis of behavior after it has occurred is not wholly reliable either, since it is often difficult for an individual to reconstruct the intuitions that lead to the selection of one option over another. Qualitative evaluation can be used to collect information on perceptions and attitudes. A focus group consisting of incoming residents can provide information on the attitudes toward the use of MEDLINE as part of the information-gathering process.

Instructor performance is crucial to the overall effectiveness of a program. Evaluation of instructor performance is an excellent way to maintain the consistency and quality of instruction. Instructors benefit from feedback on their teaching and presentation skills. Evaluation of instructors should come from three sources: the participants, the instructor, and the instructor's colleagues or supervisor. Some areas to consider when evaluating instructor performance include

- How unexpected questions, hostile audiences, equipment breakdowns, or other unforeseen events are handled.
- Whether material is delivered in a clear and concise manner.
- Poise, appearance, and presentation style of instructor.

Few graduate programs in librarianship include courses on learning theory, bibliographic instruction, and adult education [14-15], despite the recommendations of Barbara Smith's 1981 study on the educational qualifications and needs of bibliographic instruction (BI) librarians [16]. Consequently, many library school graduates have little knowledge or experience with these areas. BIS claims that over 80% of advertised academic reference positions now have BI responsibilities [17]. Thus an effort must be made to ensure that librarian educators possess effective speaking and presentation skills and a basic understanding of learning theory or cognitive learning. This effort can be aided by the evaluation process. (For further information on the preparation, recruitment, and development of staff for instruction, see Chapter 4.)

The overall value of a program should never be neglected in drawing up an evaluation agenda. This type of information is important for a variety of reasons. Often, program value must be demonstrated to administrators who know little about bibliographic instruction or who may be assessing library services. The evaluation of programs or materials can be used in the future planning of a library's user education program. Some focal points for evaluating programs include cost effectiveness, success in meeting objectives, success in meeting the needs of the intended audience, and adequacy and appropriateness of resources.

Methodologies

Once purpose, focus, and type of evaluation are determined, the next step is to select an appropriate methodology for evaluation. Evaluation methods can be divided into two categories: *quantitative* and *qualitative.*

Quantitative evaluations gather numeric data and generally proceed in a systematic way to discern relationships, collect data, and conduct statistical analyses. A relationship that might be examined is that between receiving instruction about MeSH terms and conducting successful MEDLINE searches [18]. Statistical analysis is the application of the strictures of sampling theory and the assessment of mathematical significance.

It is important since it provides reliable and reproducible measurements of a program or material.

Qualitative evaluations have a research design—that is, they look for corelationships and subjective and judgmental data—but they lack statistical analysis [19]. Although the information gathered is not subjected to the rigors of statistical analysis, qualitative evaluation can be valuable. When working with small groups, information on affective or attitudinal skills can be used to fine-tune instructional programs.

The method used, not the information obtained, determines if an evaluation is quantitative or qualitative. In other words, how the data is collected determines whether an evaluation is quantitative or qualitative.

Issues of *validity, reliability,* and *usability* must be considered regardless of the method of evaluation. *Standards for Educational and Psychological Testing* is the authoritative source for information on these issues [20].

The BIS Continuing Education Committee defines *validity* as appropriately interpreting the results of an evaluation instrument [21]. Bonnie Gratch, in *Evaluating Bibliographic Instruction,* discusses internal and external threats to validity [22]. Internal threats may include unforeseen attitudes of individual subjects in study groups. For example, if a library announces a use study of a CD-ROM product, its use might increase because a small group of patrons does not want it removed. External threats can include limiting factors such as working only with individuals who wish to cooperate in a study or who would normally spend more time doing library research [23].

Measures are *reliable* if they provide consistent and long-term indicators of the skills being learned [24]. For example, students who receive formal instruction on the use of MeSH terms can search MEDLINE more effectively than students who do not.

Usability is the ease with which a data-collection instrument can be administered, scored, and interpreted [25]. A quiz of true and false questions is easy to give, score, and interpret. The student is either right or wrong.

Examples of Quantitative Methods

There is a wide range of methodologies available for any desired evaluation. However, some of the more popular methods are not always the most reliable. Many methodologies can collect data of varying quality, depending on the skill with which they are applied.

Surveys, also known as questionnaires, are undeniably the most favored evaluation instrument [26]; however, their apparent simplicity is deceptive. Questions must be carefully constructed so that they do not influence the respondents' answers. Open-ended questions need to be constructed to allow users the opportunity to provide comments that are specific enough to provide tangible and measurable results. The survey itself should be evaluated for accuracy and content. It should be brief, to encourage higher response rates.

End-of-class feedback surveys can provide some formative evaluation information, especially surveys that ask for the learner's suggestions for change or the learner's opinion on the content and usefulness of an instructional program or handout. However, such surveys do not provide significant evaluation of higher-order skill attainment. Fatzer correctly calls them "how'm-I-doing" surveys [27.] They indicate that the respondent knows about something, but not necessarily how to do something. Such a survey might indicate that a learner knows what *Science Citation Index* is, but not how to use it. Another example of a quantitative method is tests, such as multiple choice, true-false questions, or fill in the blanks.

Examples of Qualitative Methods

Because of the complexities of collecting quantitative data and the limits on the data's usefulness, many evaluators have turned to qualitative evaluation methods when seeking to improve instructional programs.

Focus groups have become an increasingly popular method of evaluating libraries. Generally, groups of eight to twelve people will be interviewed to identify the strengths and weaknesses of library programs and services. Focus groups are usually moderated by an outsider, someone not employed by the library. Frequently, more than one focus group will be interviewed to ensure consistency in the data collected (reliability). Some of the benefits include reasonable cost, the candid information acquired, and the limited amount of time required to conduct sessions. Information from the focus groups can be useful in identifying new or changing user needs. For example, focus groups can be useful to determine if more point-of-use handouts can compensate for a reduction in instructional programs. Some drawbacks include difficulty recruiting participants (usability) and findings that cannot easily be extrapolated to a larger user population (validity). The Columbia Hospital Library in Milwaukee, Wisconsin, evaluated its services using focus group interviews. The information was used in a grant proposal for end-user technology [28].

Peer evaluation can be used for program or instructor evaluation. For program evaluation, instructional programs in one library can be compared to those in another library where the content, audience, and methods of presentation are similar. This is still a novel approach for librarians since there are usually disparities between libraries. Some differences can be assigned to the diversity of the user population, the level and quality of educational programs, and the level and quality of library skills possessed by users. Peer institutions can be found using the Association of Academic Health Sciences Library Directors (AAHSLD) statistics [29] or the *American Library Directory* [30].

When presented in a positive and uncritical manner, peer evaluation of instructors can be an enriching experience for the instructor under review. This method of evaluation provides feedback on presentation style and content. An individual's strengths and weaknesses are highlighted, and one's teaching or presentation style can be adjusted accordingly. Peer evaluation is another method of performance assessment with which library administration is beginning to experiment [31].

Interviewing is another means of achieving qualitative assessment of an instructional program or materials. This can be an expensive, time-consuming process and requires the cooperation of interviewees. Since participation is voluntary, response rates can be quite low. Interviewing can provide much of the same information as that received from focus groups. However, it does not allow interaction between the members of the user group. On the other hand, respondents are not influenced by others' responses. Effective use of interviewing methodologies requires the development of well-focused open- and close-ended questions. To reduce the costs of this methodology, interviews can be conducted by students, thereby saving professional and support staff time. Interviewers should be trained to ensure that there is quality data collection, i.e., consistency of questions and minimized bias.

Other methods exist or can be developed to collect information for evaluative purposes. In addition, many examples published in the library literature detail how libraries have implemented evaluation programs [32-34]. These case reports frequently include the positive and negative aspects of decisions made, and show how evaluations have improved programs. This type of information can be invaluable to the beginner.

Sources of Sample Instruments

Fortunately, librarians embarking on an evaluation program can obtain sample evaluation instruments from various sources. There are numerous ways to design a survey, and a novice instructor can find many good examples.

One of the most widely used sources is the Library Orientation/instruction EXchange (LOEX) Clearinghouse at Eastern Michigan University, Ypsilanti, Michigan. To use the LOEX collection, an institution must be a member of the organization. Member libraries send LOEX copies of their instructional handouts, policies, and evaluation instruments. These are then lent to other members upon request. Many libraries have modeled their handouts on those available through LOEX. The success of this clearinghouse is due to widespread cooperation by member institutions. For example, BIS directs all its samples to LOEX. (For an address, see Appendix B.)

The Educational Resources Information Centers (ERIC) collect educational materials from a wide range of sources. Many of these materials are useful to librarians. The holdings are listed in the print index, *Resources in Education*, and in the ERIC database which is available on BRS (online service now called CDP Online) and DIALOG. The items themselves can be obtained from the ERIC Document Reproduction Service or from a library that owns the microfiche collection.

Material can also be requested from the BI-L and MEDLIB-L electronic discussion lists on the Internet and BITNET networks. BI-L is an international computer conference that deals with all aspects of bibliographic instruction; MEDLIB-L focuses on all aspects of health sciences libraries and librarianship. Both electronic lists are good sources for ideas and suggestions for improving evaluation procedures. (See Appendix C.)

Looking to the Future

The Changing Environment

When well-designed and implemented, evaluation can be a valuable source of information for planning and program development. The changing environment provides the second source of information needed for creating and maintaining effective educational programs.

Every aspect of the librarian's work is subject to change. Computer technology is evolving and society will continue to take advantage of new information and communication technologies, such as electronic mail and telefacsimile. Education for the health professions is moving in new directions as problem-based curricula and computer-assisted instruction become commonplace. At the same time, health care costs are increasingly motivating health consumers to become more knowledgeable. The library profession's continuing challenge is to manage this change and exploit the opportunities it presents. To do this effectively, librarians need to understand the external forces driving change. It is always difficult to predict the future, but this section will attempt to identify trends and present models for action as health sciences librarians prepare to meet the future.

Any analysis of trends in user instruction requires a detailed look at the influences driving change. In the case of educational services, these influences will be grouped into four categories: technology, library users, the library profession, and the institutions within which health sciences librarians work.

Technology

The technologies relating to information storage, access, transfer, and management have evolved steadily. Due to the lengthy development time needed to create these products, librarians can expect opportunities for experimentation before they are widely implemented. In fact, libraries often choose to be test sites for products under development. Some of the most important of these rapidly evolving technologies are full-text, factual, and image databases; computer-assisted instruction; multimedia; and networks. Access and storage formats will become increasingly integrated to create new ways to use them. For instance, sophisticated, user-friendly front-end programs are being developed to assist users in locating and using information. Such systems provide opportunities for the design of new library tools and services. As users turn to library staff for training in the use of these tools, librarians need to be prepared to handle these responsibilities.

Much has been hypothesized about how information systems and modes of access to information will change in the twenty-first century. Clement McDonald offers some interesting scenarios [35]. He imagines computers so small that health care workers will be able to carry them as they carry beepers today. Within a similar time frame, computers will be able to accept spoken commands, thereby eliminating a long-standing barrier to use by health professionals. Data storage capabilities will improve due to inexpensive optical storage devices and, as a result, several important issues will emerge. Questions about what data to retain will diminish in importance and data management will become increasingly problematic. At the same time, retaining video images, in addition to text, becomes feasible. McDonald hypothesizes that within five years, medical information systems will contain images such as X-rays, patients' faces, electrocardiographs, and detailed illustrations such as skin lesions. Currently, the hardware and software needed to connect video cameras to computers are widely available, and their purchase price will continue to diminish. As storage costs decrease, the key factor becomes the cost of capturing data.

Fiber-optic systems available currently offer significantly more capacity than copper wires and will lower the high cost of communication. This cost reduction will foster even larger health care systems. As geographic limitations are reduced or removed, access to library services will increase in importance. With storage and communications costs reduced, users' interest and emphasis will turn to access and management issues.

Computerized decision support will have a major impact on how physicians and nurses make clinical care decisions. For example, raw clinical data will be converted to brief abstracts of basic patient care issues. Computers will provide the computational support by performing weight-dependent drug dosage analyses. Computers can also assist in selecting the best test and treatment modalities, resulting in improvement in the overall quality of care provided.

By the turn of the century, it is likely that hospitals will be allocating 10% of their budget to automation, a significant increase over the 1 to 3% spent in 1989. Most of these additional dollars will be spent on clinical information systems [36].

Given these advances in technology, the next question is: What impact will they have on the role of library-based instruction?

New Information Products

As database technology becomes increasingly sophisticated, libraries are beginning to offer end-user access to full-text and factual databases. These databases, as nonreferring sources of information, provide one-stop shopping to end users. However, users may be unprepared for the complexities of these less familiar formats.

Full-text databases offer a number of advantages to users. They free the user from coming to the library and allow multiple users simultaneous access to the same piece of information. Increased timeliness of publication may also be an eventual benefit. However, current products offer only modest gains at best. In a recent study, McKinin et al. found that BRS' Comprehensive Core Medical Library (CCML) and MEDIS offered more timely access to the literature than MEDLINE only 14% and 29% of the time, respectively [37]. Full text presents new instructional challenges as users require more sophisticated search strategies to deal with the richness and complexity of full-text searching. Users may be surprised to find that search techniques effective for bibliographic databases prove less useful when applied to full-text databases.

Like full-text databases, various types of factual databases have been used by the library community for a considerable period of time. Recently, a number of new ventures in both the private and public sectors have made these sources, and other more novel tools, widely available to end users. Some federal government agencies now offer part of the information they collect in electronic rather than print form. Examples include databases of research projects, toxic chemical release information, and some census information. (See Table 5-1.) Also, as the Human Genome Project progresses, databases comprising genetic maps and sequence information, such as the Genetic Sequences Data Bank (GenBank) [38] and the Genome Data Base (GDB) [39-40], will continue to develop and grow rapidly. Such genetic databases are currently managed by various institutions around the world. The National Center for Biotechnology Information (NCBI) is working to offer more centralized access to this type of information. One way in which NCBI is attempting to compile and disseminate information from the Human Genome Project is electronic. Through distribution of the Entrez CD-ROMs and the development of Internet accessible information services [41-42], NCBI is offering easy access to an even larger set of genome and related databases. (See Table 5-1.)

Although computerization is a powerful way to make information available, it often presents obstacles to end users. Diversity of formats, search capabilities, and connectivity problems abound. Health sciences library staff need to be prepared to assist end users in identifying, accessing, and using these rapidly growing information sources.

In addition to the publicly available factual databases being developed by the commercial and not-for-profit sectors, many institutions are creating their own in-house databases. These are comprised of local clinical records, billing information, pharmaceutical records, and similar data [43]. Increasingly, these databases will be linked by networks to other information systems. Network connections can be developed to systems like MEDLINE, full-text and factual databases, and libraries of images [44]. This arrangement offers unique opportunities for rapid access to information on a scale not previously envisioned.

Networks

Networks are the electronic links that connect computers at the local, state, regional, national, and international level. They offer the potential for developing a wide range of new technologies and services. Existing networks tie together libraries, library users, and their institutions in ways that were previously unimaginable. As more and more users learn how to take advantage of these resources, demands on the capacity of the various state, regional, and national networks will increase.

With the passage of legislation funding the National Research and Education Network (NREN), attention is focusing on the future of national networks, especially the Internet. These networks provide many users with access to new information products. By increasing the amount of information that can be transferred between computers, the NREN will increase the amount of information users can access through networks [45]. This will

Table 5-1: Examples of Factual Information Sources

DENTALPROJ
A database of research projects funded by the National Institutes of Dental Health.

TRI
Toxic Release Inventory files reporting annual toxic chemical releases. It is available on the TOXNET search system on MEDLARS.

MEDLARS Management Section
National Library of Medicine
8600 Rockville Pike
Bethesda, MD 20894
Telephone: 800-638-8480
FAX: 301-496-0822

DNA and protein sequence databases
NCBI provides access to these through the electronic mail servers: retrieve@ncbi.nlm.nih.gov and blast@ncbi.nlm.nih.gov

National Center for Biotechnology Information (NCBI)
National Library of Medicine
8600 Rockville Pike
Bethesda, MD 20894
Telephone: 301-496-2475
Internet: info@ncbi.nlm.nih.gov

1990 Census
Block maps, previously issued in paper and on microfiche, will be available only on CD-ROM or magnetic tape from NTIS, starting in 1993.

National Technical Information Service (NTIS)
U.S. Department of Commerce
Springfield, VA 22161
Telephone: 703-487-4650
FAX: 703-321-8547

Entrez: Sequences on CD-ROM
This product is a package of two CD-ROM disks: one containing MEDLINE references assigned the MeSH term, MOLECULAR SEQUENCE DATA, and the other containing molecular sequence data drawn from GenBank, PDB, PIR, SWISS-PROT, and the Protein Research Foundation.
Stock No. 717-133-00000-5 or Order No. List ID ENT

Superintendent of Documents
U.S. Government Printing Office
P.O. Box 371954
Pittsburgh, PA 15250-7954
Telephone: 202-783-3238
FAX: 202-512-2233

(For more examples of factual databases, see Volume 1 of this series: *Reference and Information Services in Health Sciences Libraries.*)

enable libraries to develop new services and reach new user groups. For instance, users might be able to send and receive video images though network connections, thus allowing the development of new forms of computer-assisted instruction for users unable or unwilling to visit the library. Currently, video information is so data intensive that network transmission on realistic time scales is impossible.

On a smaller scale, many libraries and their parent institutions are experimenting with local networks and connecting these to existing national and international networks [46]. The National Library of Medicine (NLM) sponsors efforts to connect practicing physicians with various local, regional, and national networks [47]. Currently, networks are being used for end-user searching and reference service. Experiments with document delivery are also proving promising. The Research Libraries Group (RLG) ARIEL project transmits high-quality electronic images of documents between specially equipped workstations. The project offers a new standard for transmission speed and quality [48]. In the future, high-resolution images and computer-assisted instruction may be available through networks. Increasingly, librarians are being identified as experts on networking issues, and users are turning to them for advice.

Networks provide new ways for libraries to offer their services to users, thereby eliminating some of the long-standing barriers to information access. Networks have the potential to change the way librarians relate to users. At a minimum, they will make face-to-face encounters less common. Health sciences librarians will need to devise methods for providing instruction to users whose only link to the library's services and resources will be through a network connection. Some libraries are currently meeting network-related instructional needs with classes on the use of networks and the resources they provide. As networks continue to become more widely available, demand for this type of instruction should increase. However, a dilemma results because networks create an audience of unaffiliated remote users for whom the contacted library's degree of responsibility is not entirely clear.

New Tools

In addition to new formats for obtaining and storing information, increased coordination of information technologies will improve users' options for integrating information into their decision-making processes. New tools are under development, although their final form is unclear. Several ground-breaking projects, sponsored by the National Library of Medicine, are underway at various institutions. The most prominent examples are the Unified Medical Language System (UMLS) and Integrated Advanced Information Management System (IAIMS).

Recognizing the difficulties researchers face when attempting interdisciplinary research, the NLM has made a significant long-term investment in the development of the UMLS to provide a core vocabulary common to the life sciences. This project draws from several existing health-related controlled vocabularies. The ultimate goal is the development of a single unified, but flexible, vocabulary that will allow access to the knowledge base of a wide range of disciplines. A searcher from a particular discipline will be able to use a single strategy and terminology, based on the vocabulary that is most familiar to him or her, and the UMLS will provide the capability to map the strategy for any database [49].

In addition to the UMLS, the NLM supports several academic medical centers, hospitals, and their libraries in designing new tools to access and manage information under the auspices of the IAIMS program [50]. This program seeks to promote the development of information management systems that assist health care workers in obtaining, organizing, and using medical information. The IAIMS program has produced very promising prototypes. For example, Georgetown University has developed a model system that allows medical students to combine and organize information from several sources: the medical literature, various factual databases, and patient information [51-53]. Johns Hopkins' Welch Medical Library has been working on developing parallel systems for the management of clinical information and scholarly research information [54]. Although the main focus of IAIMS to date has been at academic sites, many of the concepts can be applied at other types of information centers. Klein describes an IAIMS project at a hospital library [55]. Doubtless, similar initiatives are underway at other institutions. More will begin in the decade ahead.

At a minimum, efforts like UMLS and IAIMS will make it easier for clinicians, researchers, and others in the health professions to find and manage the information they require. Ultimately, this should lessen the need for educational services.

Computer-Assisted Instruction

As a result of increasingly integrated information storage and retrieval capabilities, computer technology offers the potential for new modes of instruction. While computer-assisted instruction (CAI) has been available for over a decade, there seems to be no dearth of ideas for new applications. A hallmark of the most recent efforts is an increasing ability to merge different types and sources of information. New developments in this area include interactive video, hypermedia, and decision support systems. For instance, factual information, images, and citations can be combined to provide support for decision making or to provide a lifelike patient simulation.

In this area, one of the most exciting advances is interactive video (IAV). It combines the branching power of the computer with video to create real-life educational opportunities. IAV accommodates the varying learning skills and styles of students, making it a particularly flexible learning media. One model for this type of instructional media is AI/LEARN, an IAV program currently available for teaching medical concepts and reasoning [56]. Taking advantage of the controlled environment provided by computer simulation, AI/LEARN offers the student a wide range of clinical experiences that may not be available at the time of need. The program teaches the student how to make accurate observations, assess the information collected, and transform it into a valid clinical decision by providing immediate or delayed feedback. AI/LEARN provides instruction in rheumatology using the knowledge base AI/RHEUM. AI/RHEUM is a database of medical facts designed to provide decision-making support to primary care physicians in diagnosing rheumatic diseases. AI/LEARN functions as a companion program to teach problem-solving and decision-making skills, one of the higher forms of cognitive learning. IAV fills a gap in traditional learning.

While evaluation of IAV programs has been limited, a study conducted at Boston University's School of Medicine provides encouraging feedback. Students who used an IAV program on trauma were highly satisfied with the learning experience. In addition, faculty believed it was a valuable learning tool that encouraged independent study, developed problem-solving skills, and stimulated further learning [57].

When hypermedia techniques are combined with IAV, a unique instructional environment is created. Hypermedia consists of color video images, sound, text, and informational databases, all of which are electronically cross-referenced and linked together. The Echocardiography Encyclopedia, developed jointly by physicians at Yale and Erasmus Universities (The Netherlands), is an example of such an application of hypermedia. The database contains information on all diseases that can be diagnosed by echocardiography. The user determines the learning sequence and level of specificity appropriate to his or her needs [58].

Another important development in the field of CAI is in the design of computer-assisted diagnosis systems. These typically use a factual knowledge base but integrate it with an inferential engine that enables users to manipulate and retrieve the information stored in the knowledge base. Rather than teaching students to use computers in the abstract, these systems require that students use computers to learn medicine. Programs include three key components: an electronic textbook, a spreadsheet to enable students to combine concepts, and an expert consultant system. The programs are intended to teach students a core body of information in a specific medical discipline.

One example of this type of program is Iliad, a computer decision support system under development at the University of Utah. It is designed for medical students in their internal medicine clerkship, as well as for house officers. The knowledge base comprises information from multiple sources including the published medical literature, patient databases, and medical specialists. In addition to offering CAI, Iliad can also function as a simulation. The user controls the instructional session, thereby providing stimulation for learning problem-solving skills and for testing progress [59].

To date, computer-assisted instruction has been a minor part of traditional library-based bibliographic instruction, even though it is widely accepted as a valid format in health sciences education. Hypertext has generated wide-ranging interest among librarians as a mechanism for incorporating CAI applications into library instruction. Its appeal stems not merely from its simplicity (applications can be developed without the aid of a software engineer), but also because it allows a multidimensional organization of information. This enables the user to branch out and explore information in ways other than the traditional linear paths of print materials. A well-designed hypertext program can offer a user access to any of several screens from any given place in the program. The user is not limited to moving page by page consecutively. The broad distribution of hypertext programs has resulted in the creation of a number of library applications, ranging from automated library tours to hypertext front ends for online catalogs. Ohio State University and the University of Denver have developed programs using hypertext to assist users in designing research strategies and using the library's online catalog [60-61].

Changing User Needs and Expectations

An entirely different type of environmental force affecting health sciences library service will be the continuing change in users' needs and expectations. As many library users become more familiar with computers and accustomed to electronic techniques for obtaining and managing information, their expectations will rise apace. At the same time, many users may be excluded from new resources and services due to fees, equipment costs, or other reasons. Some may exclude themselves from new technologies through fear and anxiety. Librarians are already experiencing conflicting demands from users. The challenge will be to balance the needs of all library users within the context of limited resources. (For a discussion of ethical decision making, see Chapter 1.)

Continuing Education

The medical community has long been aware of the spiraling growth in its information base and, as a result, continuing education (CE) has become a necessary part of health care provision. In his analysis of change in medical education, McManus predicted that medical education would shift its focus from transmitting factual information to teaching lifelong learning skills [62]. Librarians are obvious partners in the education of health care professionals throughout their careers. Health sciences librarians are beginning to recognize the contributions they can make to CE, particularly in the areas of information access and management. As academic health science libraries succeed in integrating their programs into health professions curricula, they will sow the seeds for long-term reliance on information resources.

In some cases, particularly in hospital libraries, the library itself has assumed responsibility for CE [63-64]. Even short of managing CE programs, librarians have much to contribute to the development of state-of-the-art CE. With increased emphasis on lifelong learning skills, many areas in which librarians have established expertise will be sought by practitioners. Areas such as management of electronic information sources, access to electronic forms of information, and development of current awareness plans spring to mind. Practitioners' increasing needs for up-to-date, organized, accessible clinical and research information provide a valuable opportunity for proactive information professionals. The concept of the teachable moment, described by Leist and Kristofco [65], focuses on the librarian's role in designing instructional programs that meet the immediate and specific information needs of physicians. They believe librarians can make an important contribution to clinical practice by teaching practitioners information management skills. A proactive position will be important to insure that medical libraries' parent institutions do not overlook the rich resources and valuable services that librarians make available.

Increasing Multiculturalism

Another change in health sciences libraries' user populations is increasing diversity. Librarians need to examine their attitudes and services to ensure that they are sensitive to the wide variety of cultural, ethnic, and socioeconomic backgrounds of library users. Some areas for consideration include whether to develop separate programs for users unfamiliar with libraries or computers, or for those who do not speak English as their first language. Care needs to be taken about the kind of message that will be sent to users singled out for special treatment. It is important to make these types of decisions with tact and sensitivity. Specialized instructional sessions can be oriented to users' backgrounds or skills rather than their group membership. For instance, a class could be promoted to users for whom English is a second language rather than to foreign students as a whole.

Influences within the Profession

Library Education

Not only are library users changing, so are the people staffing library desks and attending library school. In the rapidly changing profession of health sciences librarianship, individuals with advanced degrees in the sciences will be in increasing demand and of growing value to their institutions [66]. As course-integrated library instruction for health sciences students becomes the norm, such subject specialists will be poised to take a more active role in curriculum planning, development, and innovation. Furthermore, many other entry-level professionals will be skilled instructors, either through courses completed in graduate school or as a result of prior work experience. The challenge for library education will be to prepare or recruit library students who have the potential to become skilled instructors and consultants in the workplace.

Evolving Role of Librarians

As described in *Challenge to Action* [67], those health professionals possessing information-handling skills will be able to routinely integrate the latest information from a variety of disciplines with their research and clinical practice. These health professionals will become more effective in their work. To aid health care workers, librarians must assume broader roles as instructors and teach students, faculty, and practitioners the most current techniques for accessing, handling, and managing health care information [68]. Librarians will test the software and teach health care workers how to use the selected products.

In this changing environment, health sciences librarians are taking on new roles as information management professionals [69-70]. Many health sciences librarians are becoming partners in research, valued for their expertise in information access, transfer, and management.

Librarians in all health care settings may find their role as information intermediary declining in importance as end-user systems proliferate. As these systems become more widely available and heavily used, health professionals at every stage in their careers will recognize the expertise of librarians and increasingly rely on them for guidance and advice. As a result, librarians will have opportunities to take a more prominent role in carrying out the educational mission of the hospitals and academic health sciences centers in which they work. End-user instruction has opened the door for increased contact between librarians and users, but it will not be the final opportunity.

In an environment such as the one just described, librarians' long history of computer use and expertise will position them to play a major role in the strategic planning needed to successfully synthesize computer use into health care education and practice. This vision of the health sciences librarian's role corresponds with the scenarios described by Matheson and Cooper in their landmark report of 1982. The concept of IAIMS stipulates a role for librarians in managing change to the information infrastructure— the information storage, access, and management systems—at academic health sciences centers [71]. The new products and services created under the auspices of IAIMS have created new roles for librarians while also enhancing their standing among academic colleagues.

Medical Library Association Support for User Instruction

The Medical Library Association's strategic plan [72-73] spells out the organization's commitment to an instructional role for librarians. *Platform for Change,* the educational policy statement of the association, defines the knowledge and skills needed by librarians who are teaching ways to obtain, organize, and use information [74]. The organization supports the librarian's instructional role by promoting the special expertise of health sciences librarians, influencing curricular changes in library schools, recognizing professional excellence in the field, offering continuing education programs, providing assistance in identifying and funding the creation of new educational programs, and by offering referral and consultative services. Perhaps some of the association's most visible efforts have been in the area of continuing education for health sciences librarians. MLA offers courses on basic instructional techniques, working with the adult learner, and using hypermedia.

National Library of Medicine

In addition to the IAIMS and UMLS initiatives, the National Library of Medicine plays a leadership role through the development and promotion of end-user search systems such as GRATEFUL MED and document delivery systems such as LOANSOME DOC. The Learning Center for Interactive Technology is a demonstration center at NLM for clinical simulations and related teaching products. NLM also supports professional development for librarians through its train-the-trainer program. NLM convened a planning panel on the educational needs of the health sciences librarian of the future, including retraining of librarians in the work force today. In developing and testing products and services, NLM has involved a wide range of health sciences libraries and their users. Thus, the products reflect contemporary user interest and expectations. These examples emanate from NLM's goal of providing a uniform level of access to information for health care providers, regardless of their proximity to health sciences library services [75].

Influences from Parent Institutions

Pressure to Reduce the Costs of Medical Care

Cost containment will likely remain a prominent issue in the delivery of health care. Hospital librarians have made a long-term commitment to training health professionals to acquire the information they need to provide quality care at reasonable cost. Consulting the medical literature in clinical settings has been widely touted as a practice that facilitates the delivery of quality care. A recent study found that, after consulting the medical literature, 80% of the physicians studied altered the way they handled patient care [76]. Clearly there is a role for librarians in teaching health care workers how to acquire information that may lead to cost containment.

Hospitals' Efforts in Health Promotion

A related trend in hospitals is the increased interest in health promotion. Bandy describes hospital librarians' efforts to provide health information to patients and consumers [77]. Health sciences libraries have the potential to be an important resource for patient education material. To date, consumer health information has been inconsistently handled by health sciences libraries. Martin [78] and Gartenfeld [79] discuss the positive roles that health sciences librarians can play as supporters of patient educational services and providers of community health information. Others describe partnerships with public libraries in these types of efforts [80-81]. Patients often have limited information-seeking skills and limited ability to understand the literature intended for the health care provider. Librarians have an opportunity to assume a more assertive role in providing information services designed to meet the unique needs of laypeople [82-84]. (For more information on this topic, see Volume 1 of this series: *Reference and Information Services in Health Sciences Libraries.*)

The Impact of Change

The impact on library instruction from the rapidly changing environment has been painted in broad strokes thus far. It is also essential to consider the likely effect these changes will have on librarians' daily instructional activities. What is taught, how it is taught, and even who is taught will be affected. The sources of change have been discussed. Now an attempt will be made to predict the impact of these changes on the health sciences librarian's instructional role.

What Will Be Taught

As the twentieth century comes to a close, it is evident that medical education has undergone significant improvement and innovation over the past 100 years. The Flexner report in the early part of the century recommended changes that were of such significance that only now, after nearly seventy years of practice, are they being reevaluated [85]. These recent efforts confirm many of Flexner's original recommendations but also update them. In the 1984 report on the general professional education of the physician (*GPEP*) [86], prepared by the Association of American Medical Colleges, many of the recommendations made mirror those of Flexner. For example, *GPEP* recommends reducing the number of lecture hours and promoting the development of independent learning and problem-solving skills [87]. Perhaps some of the similarity can be explained by the fact that, to a significant extent, the practice of medicine is dominated by the processing, recording, retrieving, and communicating of information. With the continued exponential growth of medical information, changes in how physicians learn must take place. Recognizing this, many medical schools have implemented student-directed or problem-based curricula. These are designed to empower students to take responsibility for their education, rather than attempting the impossible task of teaching students all the information they will need for their medical careers. To help students master the factual content of the medical curriculum, many institutions are using computer-based simulations (some of which were described earlier) to promote the development of problem-solving skills.

For example, at Harvard Medical School, information technologies are integrated into the curriculum. As a result, computer usage has become an ordinary routine in the practice of medicine. The computer is viewed as a tool that will promote self-teaching and encourage the acquisition of skills needed to seek information, test hypotheses, and contribute to the creation of new knowledge. To date, the use of information technologies in the Harvard curriculum has focused on four areas: knowledge access, including bibliographic database searching; patient and physiologic simulations; integration of graphics and video images for the study of the body's organs; and the creation of a clinical case book for each of the patients for whom the student is responsible (medical record keeping) [88]. Particularly in the area of knowledge access, the Countway Library has been actively involved in implementing this new vision of the medical curriculum.

Another example of what librarians can contribute to the information management education of health professionals is illustrated by the approach adopted at the University of Calgary. There, information management has been integrated into the medical school curriculum, not as a course, but as a repeated theme throughout the curriculum. This approach resulted from the belief that the ability to practice and develop information management skills is central to a successful career as a physician. Learning these skills at the outset and practicing them throughout the undergraduate medical program encourages the development of self-directed, independent learning styles. Other traditional horizontal themes that exist in most medical school curricula include pathology, biochemistry, and gross anatomy. The following components are introduced in sequential order into the curriculum at the University of Calgary: word processing, computer-aided learning, and electronic mail. In the future, students will have an opportunity to work with artificial intelligence systems. Throughout, the planning team included the directors of the learning resource center and the medical library [89].

Medical students are not the only health professionals benefiting from the integration of information technologies into the curriculum. Sparks reports on the instructional uses of computers in nursing education at all levels [90]. Culling from the published literature, she documents a wide range of uses. While CAI programs are the most prevalent, approximately 20% of nursing instructional programs are using computers to teach basic subjects such as nutrition, pediatric and maternal nursing, and drug solution calculation. Perusal of *Computers in Nursing* attests to nursing educators' increasing interest in integrating computer technology into the curriculum. While medical schools are clearly the innovators in using information technologies, other health professions are following this lead.

As these examples suggest, what the librarian teaches will continue to be heavily influenced by the needs of the library's immediate users. These needs vary somewhat because of differences in each institution's mission and environment. In some settings, such as highly focused research institutions, subject-oriented instruction will become very important, because the knowledge base of biomedicine is increasingly interdisciplinary. In other settings, teaching generic information management and problem-solving skills will enable users to pursue lifelong learning. As the body of knowledge in most biomedical science disciplines increases, it will be important for users to learn how to evaluate and sort the information they have retrieved so that it can be easily managed and manipulated. To support this enhanced instructional role, librarians will need to understand not only the systems and technology that will provide the course material but also how adults learn [91].

How Users Will Be Taught

As electronic communication systems become more widely accepted and more heavily used, librarians will be under significant pressure to develop services and skills to effectively communicate with users whom they rarely meet face-to-face. At one time or another, many different users are likely to fit this category. The faculty member on sabbatical, the third-year medical student doing a clinical clerkship at an affiliated hospital 200 miles away, community-based practices, and referring physicians are all potential remote users. Advances in telecommunications and remote access to local area networks make it increasingly easy to provide a range of services to these users. However, the need for off-site training will accompany the availability of these services. It will be necessary to conduct one-on-one tutorials or even group instruction in an electronic mode. As a ground-breaking example of this type of network-facilitated instruction, Internet users were offered a course, "Navigating the Internet: an Interactive Workshop," provided by Richard Smith, a librarian [92]. The entire course, including registration, was conducted by electronic mail. It will be important for librarians to acquire the skills that will help them succeed in such a highly automated environment.

Tools such as interactive video and hypermedia will enable librarians to create instructional aids. As the campus experts on information retrieval, librarians need to assume responsibility for identifying the information for specialized knowledge bases. When systems use existing graphic materials, librarians, through their knowledge of the medical literature, could select the materials. Librarians with advanced scientific training or computing skills will work in close collaboration with academic faculty to analyze curricular needs and create instructional IAV programs that will revolutionize education for the health professions [93]. Through their close contact with end users, librarians will be in an excellent position to diagnose system deficiencies and to work with system designers to make needed improvements.

The INTERNIST-1/QMR program is an excellent model for this type of expanded role for librarians. Under development at the University of Pittsburgh, QMR's knowledge base contained information on 600 diseases in internal medicine by the late 1980s. Ultimately, the program will be able to produce instantaneous summaries of articles that meet the requester's unique needs, while providing access to the full text of original articles. In a unique collaboration, a librarian, while a medical student at the University of Pittsburgh, created and stored the MeSH terminology used to search the MEDLINE database for each of the diseases in the QMR knowledge base. It will not be necessary for librarians to attend medical school to collaborate on such projects in the future, but it will be critical for them to be integral members of the research and development team [94].

Who Will Be Taught

Changing technology and advancing telecommunications systems have made the health sciences library increasingly accessible to less traditional users such as staff in remote locations, on-site staff who rarely use health sciences libraries, multidisciplinary researchers, and health services consumers. These new users have different backgrounds, experiences, and needs, and provide new challenges for information service providers.

Today's satellite connections make the hospital accessible even when the physician is hundreds of miles away. As physicians become more computer literate, they will seek remote access to hospital and academic information systems. Already, many physicians can access patient records, accounts receivable, and informational databases through a simple telephone connection. In the future, they will be able to obtain up-to-the-minute status reports on patients' conditions from remote locations. While many of these developments are not directly relevant to library systems, they provide a platform that could include gateways to library databases and other information resources and services. Librarians need to be prepared to make information available to all affiliated physicians, regardless of their location. In addition, the National Library of Medicine has mandated outreach to unaffiliated and underserved health professionals [95].

Currently, use of telefacsimile equipment is serving the information needs of remote users. As information systems become more sophisticated, librarians need to become increasingly adept at remote interviewing so that they can identify users' needs and meet them [96]. Remote users have been described as demanding, with high expectations, and frequently needing hand-holding and reassurance. It will be important to select staff who are patient and able to offer additional assistance to this new category of user [97].

To date, technology has had the most significant impact on physicians, but its impact is being felt in other health sciences disciplines as well. A case in point is the interest in nursing informatics and the development in the late 1980s of advanced degree programs in informatics for nurses. Pharma-

Administration of Educational Services

Elizabeth H. Wood

Administering a systematic user education program can be a daunting task. When a health sciences library considers any kind of teaching program, a number of issues arise: users' needs, the target audience, staffing, teacher training, special equipment, space, advertising, costs. In a one-person library, the librarian may have difficulty finding the time or resources to manage a program and may also lack the encouragement and assistance of colleagues or co-workers. Staff in a large academic library, who want to initiate an ambitious program for their many and varied users, may be overwhelmed by the logistics of organizing schedules, teachers, and materials.

This chapter covers management of educational programs and includes the topics of marketing, staffing, staff development, and support. Management of microcomputer centers and learning labs is also discussed at length because of the significant investment of time and money these special teaching facilities require. Suggestions are provided that will suit libraries of different types and sizes. In addition, the chapter reflects the needs of various library users, such as physicians, allied health professionals, students, and the administrative staff of hospitals and academic units.

Marketing

Health sciences libraries are typically nonprofit or nonrevenue producing departments within their institutions. Even so, the concept of marketing cists have been information professionals and critical members of the health care team for some time—accessing, interpreting, and evaluating drug information in collaboration with physicians. Now that many hospitals have mounted electronic versions of important drug information tools on their mainframe computers, librarians may come under additional pressure to provide training in the use of these tools.

As multidisciplinary research is encouraged on many university campuses, researchers with little previous experience in the biomedical sciences will be collaborating with health scientists. These collaborators will need basic skills training covering the organization of the medical literature and how to assess the validity of data in research fields in which they lack formal training.

As discussed earlier, patients are now increasingly interested in health information. As patients become more aware of their own health and healthful practices, health sciences libraries will be under pressure to provide a wider range of services to them, including educational services. This will be especially true of hospital libraries. Health consumers may prove to be the group providing the greatest challenge to librarians due to the diversity of their needs and backgrounds and the degree to which they require special services [98].

Librarians will need to develop educational services and teaching methods to meet the diverse needs of health information users, while bearing in mind the variety of technological comfort levels that these users bring with them. This expanded demand for instruction could place a heavy burden on librarians and may signal the need for an enhanced instructional role for support staff. These library staff members could be trained to become responsible for most basic skills training. Another way to meet new pressures may be to use artificial intelligence to make systems more intuitive and user-friendly. Also, computer-aided learning can free librarians from personally supervising many end users' instructional sessions. These and other creative strategies will be needed to meet the increasing instructional demands confronting health sciences library staff.

Summary

Several themes emerge from the preceding analysis. Information will be increasingly easy and inexpensive to access and store and will result in a rapid proliferation of new information products and applications. Some of the most exciting developments will result from efforts to integrate various sources and media to develop completely new ways to manage and use information. Many of the dilemmas described above result from attempting to graft new technology onto existing service patterns. Perhaps part of the solution lies in developing completely new services. Matheson and Cooper [99] point out that evolving technologies are typically used initially for replacement—doing an old task more efficiently—and only later are they transformational, enabling the development of completely new services. The challenge librarians will face is envisioning and developing technologies to create new, easy-to-use, and more effective services.

Perhaps the best example of this is the vision of the virtual library. Mitchell and Saunders describe the virtual library as providing access to all the services and resources of the library at the user's desktop [100]. Current technologies are beginning to make this possible as networks provide remote connections to libraries. Librarians and library users are beginning to transform the way information is organized and used.

Finally, librarians will take on new roles in their relations with their users. The greatest benefits of this change will result if librarians work closely with knowledge engineers to develop new technologies, yet maintain a strong grasp of users' needs. Instruction will provide an important vehicle for expanding the relationship between librarians and health sciences professionals.

References

1. Schlichter D, Pemberton J. The Emperor's new clothes? Problems of the user survey as a planning tool in academic libraries. Coll Res Libr 1992 May;53(5):257-265.

2. Research Committee's Subcommittee on Evaluation. Bibliographic Instruction Section. Association of College and Research Libraries. American Library Association. Evaluating bibliographic instruction: a handbook. Chicago: Association of College and Research Libraries, 1983.

3. Bloom BS et al. Taxonomy of educational objectives. Handbook I: Cognitive objectives. New York: David McKay, 1956.

4. Ibid., 7.

5. Hernon P, McClure CR. Evaluation and library decision making. Norwood, NJ: Ablex, 1990.

6. Hardesty L. Evaluation of bibliographic instruction. Presented to the Alabama Library Instruction Roundtable, Alabama Library Association. 9 April 1986. (ERIC document no. 271115.)

7. Ibid., 7.

8. Ibid.

9. Hernon, op. cit, 5.

10. Continuing Education Committee. Bibliographic Instruction Section. Association of College and Research Libraries. Organizing and managing a library instruction program checklists. Rev. ed. 1986. (ERIC document no. 294596.)

11. Werking RH. Evaluating bibliographic education: a review and critique. Libr Trends 1980 Summer;29(1):153-172.

12. Hardesty, op. cit., 10.

13. Fatzer JB. Evaluation of library user instruction. RQ 1987 Fall;27(1):41-43.

14. Patterson CD, Howell DW. Library user education: assessing the attitudes of those who teach. RQ 1990 Summer;29(2):513-523.

15. Mandernack S. An assessment of education and training needs for bibliographic instruction librarians. J Educ Libr Inf Sci 1990 Winter;30(3):193-205.

16. Smith BJ. Background characteristics and education needs of a group of instruction librarians in Pennsylvania. Coll Res Libr 1982 May;43(5):197-207.

17. Grassian E. More on BIS Task Force. Message to: BI-L. In BI-L [BITNET/Internet listserv]. Raish M, list owner. Binghamton: State University of New York at Binghamton, 1992 Nov 16, 10:58 [61 lines].

18. Hardesty, op. cit., 18.

19. Ibid.

20. Committee to Develop Standards for Educational and Psychological Testing of the American Educational Research Association. American Psychological Association and the National Council on Measurement in Education. Standards for educational and psychological testing. Washington, DC: American Psychological Association, 1985.

21. Continuing Education Committee. Bibliographic Instruction Section, op.cit., 19.

22. Gratch BG. Research designs appropriate for evaluating bibliographic instruction. In: Evaluating bibliographic instruction: a handbook. Chicago: American Library Association, 1983:37-60.

23. Ibid.

24. Hardesty, op. cit., 23.

25. Continuing Education Committee. Bibliographic Instruction Section, op. cit., 19.

26. Werking, op. cit., 162.

27. Fatzer, op. cit., 42.

28. Robbins K, Holst R. Hospital library evaluation using focus group interviews. Bull Med Libr Assoc 1990 Jul;78(3):311-313.

29. Association of Academic Health Sciences Library Directors. Annual statistics of medical school libraries in the United States and Canada. 14th ed. Houston: Association of Academic Health Sciences Library Directors, 1992.

30. American library directory. New York: R.R. Bowker, 1923-.

31. Reifler H. Peer evaluation at Washington State University Libraries: a two-year experiment. J Libr Admin 1983 Summer;4(2):51-73.

32. Tiefel V. Evaluating a library user education program: a decade of experience. Coll Res Libr 1989 Mar;50(3):249-259.

33. Kenney PA, McArthur JN. Designing and evaluating a programmed library instruction text. Coll Res Libr 1984 Jan;45(1):35-42.

34. Sugranes MP, Neal JA. Evaluation of a self-paced bibliographic instruction course. Coll Res Libr 1983 Nov;44(6):444-457.

35. McDonald CJ. Medical information systems of the future. MD Comput 1989 Mar/Apr;6(2):82-7.

36. Ibid., 86.

37. McKinin EJ, Sievert M, Collins BR. Currency of full-text medical journals: CCML and MEDLINE. Bull Med Libr Assoc 1991 Jul;79(3):282-287.

38. Benson D, Lipman DJ, Ostell J. GenBank. Nucleic Acids Res 1993 Jul 1; 21(13):2963-5.

39. Cuticchia AJ et al. The GDB Human Genome Database Anno 1993. Nucleic Acids Res 1993 Jul 1; 21(13):3003-6.

40. Brandt KA. The GDB Human Genome Data Base: a source of integrated genetic mapping and disease data. Bull Med Libr Assoc 1993 Jul;81(3):285-92.

41. NCBI Continues GenBank Services. NCBI News 1992 Sep; 1(3):1-2.

42. Woodsmall RM, Benson DA. Information resources at the National Center for Biotechnology Information. Bull Med Libr Assoc 1993 Jul;81(3):282-4.

43. Stead WW. Systems for the year 2000: the case for an integrated database. MD Comput 1991 Mar/Apr;8(2):103-4.

44. National Library of Medicine. Long range plan. Report of panel 3. Obtaining factual information from data bases. Bethesda, MD: National Institutes of Health, 1986.

45. Fisher S. Whither NREN? Byte 1991 Jul;16(7):181-6,188-9.

46. Kittle PW. Networking the light fantastic—CD-ROMs on LANs. CD-ROM Prof 1992 Jan;5(1):30-31.

47. National Library of Medicine. Long range plan. Report of panel 2. Locating and gaining access to medical and scientific literature. Bethesda, MD: National Institutes of Health, 1986.

48. Jackson ME. Using ARIEL, RLG's document transmission system to improve document delivery in the United States. Interlend Doc Supply 1992 Apr;20(2):49-52.

49. Humphreys BL, ed. Symposium: The unified medical language system: current research and development. Bull Med Libr Assoc 1993 Apr;81(2):169-222.

50. Lorenzi NM, ed. Symposium: a decade of IAIMS. Bull Med Libr Assoc 1992 Jul;80(3):240-93.

51. Broering NC. The MAClinical workstation project at Georgetown University. Bull Med Libr Assoc 1991 Jul;79(3):276-81.

52. Broering NC, Corn M, Ayers WR, Mistry P. Implementing RECONSIDER, a diagnostic prompting computer system, at the Georgetown University Medical Center. Bull Med Libr Assoc 1988 Apr;76(2):155-8.

53. Broering NC, Hylton JS, Guttmann R, Eskridge D. BioSYNTHESIS: access to a knowledge network of health sciences databases. J Med Syst 1991 Apr;15(2):139-53.

54. Matheson NW, Lucier RE, Reynolds RE, Butter KA. Johns Hopkins University, Welch Medical Library. In: Arms C, ed. Campus strategies for libraries and electronic information. Bedford, MA: Digital Equipment Corporation, 1990:275-304.

55. Klein MS. Adapting IAIMS to a hospital library level. Bull Med Libr Assoc 1989 Oct;77(4):357-65.

56. Mitchell JA et al. AI/Learn: an interactive videodisk system for teaching medical concepts and reasoning. J Med Syst 1987 Dec;11(6):421-9.

57. Cullbert AJ, Jr, Cantelmo NL, Stafford ME, Allan DM. Interactive videodisc as an instructional tool in medical education. Methods Inf Med 1989 Nov;28(4):357-9.

58. Jaffee CC, Lynch PJ, Smeulders AW. Hypermedia techniques for diagnostic imaging instruction: videodisk echocardiography encyclopedia. Radiology 1989 May;171(2):475-80.

59. Warner HR, Jr. Iliad: moving medical decision-making into new frontiers. Methods Inf Med 1989 Nov;28(4):370-2.

60. Tiefel V. The gateway to information: a system redefines how libraries are used. Am Libr 1991 Oct;22(9):858-60.

61. Tschanz V. Assessment of a HyperCard program at Penrose Library, University of Denver. Ref Serv Rev 1991 Spring;19(2):39-47.

62. McManus IC. How will medical education change? Lancet 1991 Jun 22;337(8756):1519-1521.

63. Messerle J. The changing continuing education role of health sciences libraries. Bull Med Libr Assoc 1990 Apr;78(2):180-187.

64. Doyle JD, Wellik KE. Information and educational services. In: Holst R, ed. Hospital library management. 2d ed. Metuchen, NJ: Medical Library Association and Scarecrow Press. In preparation.

65. Leist JC, Kristofco RE. The changing paradigm for continuing medical education: impact of information on the teachable moment. Bull Med Libr Assoc 1990 Apr;78(2):173-9.

66. Glasgow VL, Foreman G. Subject expertise among MEDLINE searchers: results of a survey and analysis of job openings. Bull Med Libr Assoc 1984 June;72(3):257-261.

67. Joint Task Force of the Association of Academic Health Sciences Library Directors and the Medical Library Association. Challenge to action: planning and evaluation guidelines for academic health sciences libraries. Chicago: Association of Academic Health Sciences Library Directors and the Medical Library Association, 1987.

68. Ibid., 16.

69. Shipman BL, Schwartz DG, Dow SC. End user searching and new roles for librarians. Med Ref Serv Q 1992 Fall;11(3):1-16.

70. Schwartz DG. New roles for the medical librarian in an information management environment. Med Ref Serv Q 1987 Winter;6(4):27-33.

71. Matheson N, Cooper JAD. Academic information in the academic health sciences center: roles for the library in information management. J Med Educ 1982 Oct;57(part 2)10:1-93.

72. Shaping the future: the strategic plan of the Medical Library Association, 1989 revision. MLA News 1989 Jun/Jul;(216):15-26.

73. Shaping the future: the strategic plan of the Medical Library Association. MLA News 1987 Apr;(196):s1-s16

74. Medical Library Association. Platform for change: the educational policy statement of the Medical Library Association. Chicago: Medical Library Association, [1991]:[16].

75. National Library of Medicine. Long range plan. Report of panel 2, op. cit., 8.

76. Marshall JG. The impact of the hospital library on clinical decision making: the Rochester study. Bull Med Libr Assoc 1992 Apr;80(2):169-178.

77. Bandy M. Health information for patients and consumers. In: Holst R, ed. Hospital library management. 2d ed. Chicago: Medical Library Association. In preparation.

78. Martin RM. Library and health information services for patients. In: Bradley J, Holst R, Messerle J, eds. Hospital library management. Chicago: Medical Library Association, 1983.

79. Gartenfeld E. Community access to health information. In: Bradley J, Holst R, Messerle J, eds. Hospital library management. Chicago: Medical Library Association, 1983.

80. Lansing PS, Tooey MJ. Making a difference: partnerships with public libraries. Paper presented at the annual meeting of the Medical Library Association. Washington, DC. May 15-21, 1992.

81. Rees AM, ed. Managing consumer health information services. Phoenix, AZ: Oryx, 1991.

82. Arcari RD, Richetelle AL. Healthnet: Connecticut Consumer Health Information Network: an administrative and operational perspective. In: Rees AM, ed. Managing consumer health information services. Phoenix, AZ: Oryx, 1991:39-58.

83. Reidelbach MA, Weaver CG, Epperson BK. CHIRS: Consumer Health Information Resources for Nebraska residents. In: Rees AM, ed. Managing consumer health information services. Phoenix, AZ: Oryx, 1991:59-72.

84. LaRocco A. The Ellen Gartenfeld Health Information Network (EGHIN). In: Rees AM, ed. Managing consumer health information services. Phoenix: Oryx, 1991:73-82.

85. Bussigel MN, Barzansky BM, Grenholm GG. Innovation processes in medical education. New York: Praeger, 1988.

86. Association of American Medical Colleges. Physicians for the twenty-first century: report of the project panel on the general professional education of the physician and college preparation for medicine. J Med Educ 1984 Nov;59(11) Part 2:1-208.

87. Ibid., 11-12.

88. Barnett O. Information technology and undergraduate medical education. Acad Med 1989 Apr;64(4):187-90.

89. Jennett PA et al. Preparing our physicians for tomorrow—information management as a theme in undergraduate medical education. In: van Bemmel JH, Zvarova J, eds. Knowledge, information and medical education. Amsterdam: Elsevier, 1991.

90. Sparks SN. Computer-based education in nursing. Bethesda, MD: National Library of Medicine, Lister Hill National Center for Biomedical Communications, Educational Technology Branch, 1990.

91. Stoffle CJ. Public services of the future: future roles for librarians. In: Kusnerz PA, ed. The architecture library of the future: complexity and contradiction. Ann Arbor: University of Michigan, 1989.

92. On Line. Chron Higher Ed 1992 Nov 11;39(12):A19.

93. Rizzolo MA. Factors influencing the development and use of interactive video in nursing education: a Delphi study. Comput Nurs 1990 Jul-Aug;8(4):151-9.

94. Miller RA, Masarie FE, Jr. Use of the Quick Medica Reference (QMR) program as a tool for medical education. Methods Inf Med 1989 Nov;28(4):340-5.

95. National Library of Medicine. Improving health professionals' access to information: report of the Board of Regents. Bethesda, MD: U.S. Department of Health and Human Services, National Institutes of Health, 1989.

96. Wilkinson R. Making friends with MDs via telecommunications. Hospitals 1988 Jan 5;62(1):54,56-7.

97. Kalin SW. Support services for remote users of online public access catalogs. RQ 1991 Winter;31(2):197-213.

98. Bandy, op. cit. In preparation.

99. Matheson, op. cit., 2.

100. Mitchell M, Saunders LM. The virtual library: an agenda for the 1990s. Comput Libr 1991 Apr;11(4):8-11.

Appendix A

Selected List of Organizations Offering Help with Presentation Techniques

ACRL/BIS Continuing Education Committee
c/o American Library Association
50 E. Huron Street
Chicago, IL 60611
Telephone: 800-545-2433

Headquarters Library and Information Center (ext. 2153) can provide a brochure describing ALA's continuing education offerings.

American Society for Training and Development
Box 1443
1640 King Street
Alexandria, VA 22313
Telephone: 703-683-8100
FAX: 703-683-8103

Fred Pryor Seminars
2000 Shawnee Mission Parkway
Shawnee Mission, KS 66205
Telephone: 800-255-6139

National Society for Performance and Instruction
1300 L Street NW, Suite 1250
Washington, DC 20005
Telephone: 202-408-7969
FAX: 202-408-7972

Professional Development Section
c/o Special Libraries Association
1700 18th Street, N.W.
Washington, DC 20009-2508
Telephone: 202-234-4700

Toastmasters International
P.O. Box 9052
Mission Viejo, CA 92690
Telephone: 714-858-8255

Appendix B

Sources of Instructional Materials

ACRL Bibliographic Instruction Section (BIS)
BIS Newsletter
c/o ALA/ACRL
50 E. Huron Street
Chicago, IL 60611
Telephone: 800-545-2433

Library Instruction Round Table News
American Library Association
50 E. Huron Street
Chicago, IL 60611
Telephone: 800-545-2433

LOEX Clearinghouse
University Library
Eastern Michigan University
Ypsilanti, MI 48197
Telephone: 313-487-0168
FAX: 313-487-8861 (Attn: LOEX)

Public Services Section
General Reference SIG
c/o Medical Library Association
Six North Michigan Avenue, Suite 300
Chicago, IL 60602-4805
Telephone: 312-419-9094

The Public Services Section also has an Information Management Education Special Interest Group (IME SIG).

WILU (Workshop on Instruction in Library Use)
c/o Bob Elliott
Leddy Library
University of Windsor
Windsor, Ontario N9B 3P4
Canada
Telephone: 519-253-4232 Ext. 3161
FAX: 519-973-7076 (Attn: WILU, Bob Elliott)

This annual Canadian workshop, which features a sharing session on instructional materials, is held in different locations.

Appendix C

Electronic Discussion Lists

BI-L (bibliographic instruction)
BITNET: BI-L@BINGVMB.BITNET
Internet: BI-L%BINGVMB.BITNET@CUNYVM.CUNY.EDU

For more information contact

Martin Raish
Box 6012, Main Library
University at Binghamton
Binghamton, NY 13902-6012
Telephone: 607-777-4385
BITNET: MRAISH%BINGVMB.BITNET@UGA.CC.UGA.EDU

BIBSOFT (bibliographic database management)
BITNET: BIBSOFT@INDYCMS.BITNET
Internet: BIBSOFT@INDYCMS.IUPUI.EDU

For more information contact

James Morgan
Ruth Lilly Medical Library
Indiana University School of Medicine
975 W. Walnut
Indianapolis, IN 46202
Telephone: 317-274-1408
FAX: 317-274-2088
Internet: MORGANJ@INDYVAX.IUPUI.EDU

OR

Sue E. Stigleman
P.O. Box 8074
Asheville, NC 28814-8074
Telephone: 704-251-9059
Internet: STIGLE@CS.UNCA.EDU

MEDLIB-L (medical libraries)
BITNET: MEDLIB-L@UBVM.BITNET
Internet: MEDLIB-L@UBVM.CC.BUFFALO.EDU

For more information contact

Nancy Start
Health Sciences Library
University at Buffalo
Buffalo, NY 14214
Telephone: 716-831-3337
BITNET: HSLSTART@UBVM
Internet: HSLSTART@UBVM.CC.BUFFALO.EDU

PACS-L (public-access computer systems)
Internet: PACS-L@UHUPVM1.UH.EDU

For more information contact

Jill Hackenberg
University Libraries
University of Houston
Houston, TX 77204-2091
Telephone: 713-743-9761
Internet: LIBJ@JETSON.UH.EDU

OR

Dana Rooks
University Libraries
University of Houston
Houston, TX 77204-2091
Telephone: 713-743-9807
Internet: LIBL@UHUPVM1.UH.EDU

OR

Linda Thompson
University Libraries
University of Houston
Houston, TX 77204-2091
Telephone: 713-743-9808
Internet: LIB1J@UHUPVM1.UH.EDU

For information on subscribing or using these and related lists see:

Mikita EG, Drusedum LA. Introducing health sciences librarians to the Internet. Med Ref Serv Q 1993 Fall;12(3):1-12.

Okerson A, ed. Directory of electronic journals, newsletters and academic discussion lists. 4th ed. Washington, DC:Association of Research Libraries, 1994.

Raish M. BI-L: an electronic discussion group for IME. Med Ref Serv Q 1992 Summer;11(2):79-88.

Glossary

AAHSLD	Association of Academic Health Sciences Library Directors
ACRL	Association of College and Research Libraries
ALA	American Library Association
ARIEL	Document transmission system (The Research Libraries Group, Inc.)
AVLINE	Audiovisuals Online (database—NLM)
BI	Bibliographic instruction
BIBSOFT	Bibliographic database management discussion list on the Internet
BI-L	Bibliographic instruction discussion list on the Internet
BIS	Bibliographic Instruction Section (ALA)
BITNET	Because It's Time NETwork
BRS	Bibliographic Retrieval Services (online service now called CDP Online)
CAI	Computer-assisted instruction
CAR	Computer-Aided Reference station (University of Tennessee at Memphis)
CBT	Computer-based training
CCML	Comprehensive Core Medical Library (database—BRS)
CD-ROM	Compact Disk, Read-Only Memory
CE	Continuing education
CINAHL	*Cumulative Index to Nursing and Allied Health Literature*
CML	Clinical medical librarian
DIALOG	Online search service (Dialog Information Services, Inc.)
EGAD	Electronic Guide And Directory (University of Maryland at Baltimore)
ERIC	Educational Resources Information Centers
FAX	Telefacsimile
GDB	Genome Data Base (database—NLM)
GenBank	Genetic Sequences Data Bank (database—NLM)
GPEP	*General Professional Education of the Physician*
GRATEFUL MED	User-friendly microcomputer based software for searching the MEDLARS system (NLM)

IAIMS	Integrated Advanced Information Management System (was formerly Integrated Academic Information Management System)
IAV	Interactive video
ILL	Interlibrary loan
Internet	Network of networks using Standard Telecommunications Protocol
IME	Information management education
KWIC	Key word in context
KWOC	Key word out of context
LAN	Local area network
LATCH	Literature Attached to the CHart
LCD	Liquid crystal display
LITA	Library and Information Technology Association
LOANSOME DOC	Document ordering feature of the GRATEFUL MED software (NLM)
LOEX	Library Orientation/instruction EXchange
LSI	Learning style instrument
MEDIS	MEDical Information System (database—Mead Data Central)
MEDLARS	MEDical Literature Analysis and Retrieval System (NLM)
MEDLIB-L	Medical libraries discussion list on the Internet
MEDLINE	MEDLARS OnLine (database—NLM)
MEDSTATS	MEDical STATistics (expert system—NLM)
MeSH	*Medical Subject Headings*
MLA	Medical Library Association
NCBI	National Center for Biotechnology Information
NLM	National Library of Medicine
NREN	National Research and Education Network
OASIS	Online Access System for Information Sources (University of Iowa)
OCLC	Online Computer Library Center
OPAC	Online public access catalog
PACS-L	Public-access computer systems discussion list on the Internet
PC	Personal computer
PSS	Public Services Section (MLA)
RLG	Research Libraries Group
SCAMC	Symposium on Computer Applications in Medical Care
SIG	Special interest group
SME	Subject matter expert

UMABnet	Gopher system (University of Maryland at Baltimore)
UMLS	Unified Medical Language System (NLM)
WAIS	Wide area information service

Index

This is primarily a subject index. Personal authors of references cited in the text are not indexed. Acronyms and initialisms are given preference as indexing terms if more commonly used than full names of organizations or publications.

Author Biographies

Francesca Allegri was Head of Information Management Education Services at the Health Sciences Library, University of North Carolina at Chapel Hill from 1985 to 1989. From 1989 to 1991, she was Adjunct Faculty and Visiting Assistant Professor, Graduate School of Library and Information Science, University of Illinois at Urbana-Champaign. Currently, she is a consultant in the areas of in-service training and user education. She has taught and written extensively on library instruction topics.

Karla Hahn is currently Network-based Services Manager at the William H. Welch Medical Library, where previously she was the Manager for Curriculum Support. Her experiences in medical libraries includes participation in the University of Michigan Library Residency Program, where she worked in all three campus health sciences libraries.

Abigail Hubbard was Director of Education at the HAM-TMC Library at the Texas Medical Center in Houston from 1984 to 1988, where she introduced proactive information management education programs for health sciences faculty and students and published and lectured extensively about client-centered education. Current commitments include management consulting in the area of change and productivity improvement, and teaching in the MBA program at the University of Houston. In addition, she conducts numerous continuing education seminars for corporate and nonprofit sector clients, including libraries and professional library associations.

Nadia J. Martin is Reference/Instructional Librarian at the Undergraduate Library of the University of Michigan. She is also an online searcher for Advanced Information Consultants, a fee-based service for private companies. Previously she was an Information Services Librarian at the Alfred Taubman Medical Library of the University of Michigan, where she was actively involved in all aspects of education for on-site and remote users of electronic health sciences information.

Diane G. Schwartz was a medical librarian at the Alfred Taubman Medical Library, University of Michigan, from 1978 to 1992, where her responsibilities included Coordinator, Health Sciences Information Services; Head, Reference/Information Services; and Coordinator, User Education. At the University of Michigan, her interests focused on integrating instruction in the use of information technologies into the curricula of the schools of Medicine, Nursing, and Pharmacy, while ensuring that faculty from each of these schools also had the opportunity to develop their skills in this arena. Currently at the University at Buffalo, she is responsible for developing programs to teach academic primary care physicians the skills needed to become effective instructors and researchers. She is also working to develop model academic training sites which will provide primary care residents and faculty with state-of-the-art facilities for accessing, using, and managing information.

Mary Joan (M.J.) Tooey has been at the Health Sciences Library, University of Maryland at Baltimore, since 1986, where she began her services as the Head of Information Management Education. Currently, she is the Director of Information and Instructional Services, which includes the reference, searching, computer user, and education services of the Library. Her background also includes five years as a hospital librarian. She served as a delegate to the second White House Conference on Libraries and Information Services. She is also the editor of the Information Management Education column for *Medical Reference Services Quarterly.*

Melanie L. Wilson has been involved in user education since 1981. She has held appointments in academic medical libraries in information services and collection management and served as User Education Coordinator for the Norris Medical Library at the University of Southern California. There she also served as information consultant for a problem-based learning group in the School of Medicine. Along with faculty colleagues at the University of Illinois, she helped to found the College of Medicine's first critical review course for medical students. She has authored and presented papers on user education and information services.

Elizabeth H. Wood is Head of Reference at the University of Southern California (USC) Norris Medical Library, which has one of the most extensive user education programs in the country. She has taught a variety of information management and computer literacy classes—at USC, on a consultant basis for health professionals, and at regional and national Medical Library Association meetings. She has written articles and book chapters about computer literacy, teaching information management, and implementing CD-ROM searching. She is also editor of the From the Literature column for *Medical Reference Services Quarterly.*